Exercise Prescription

A Case Study Approach to the ACSM Guidelines

David P. Swain, PhD
Brian C. Leutholtz, PhD
Old Dominion University

WITHDRAWN

Library of Congress Cataloging-in-Publication Data

Swain, David P.
   Exercise prescription : a case study approach to the ACSM guidelines / David P. Swain, Brian C. Leutholtz.
      p. cm.
   Includes bibliographical references and index.
   ISBN 0-7360-3754-3
      1. Exercise therapy--Case studies.   I. Leutholtz, Brian C. II. Title.

RM725 .S92 2001
615.8'2--dc21

2001039458

ISBN: 0-7360-3754-3

Acquisitions Editor: Michael S. Bahrke, PhD; **Developmental Editor:** Jennifer Clark; **Managing Editor:** Amy Stahl; **Assistant Editors:** Derek Campbell and Amanda Gunn; **Copyeditor:** Brian Mustain; **Proofreader:** Sarah Wiseman; **Indexer:** Marie Rizzo; **Permission Manager:** Dalene Reeder; **Graphic Designer:** Fred Starbird; **Graphic Artist:** Denise Lowry; **Cover Designer:** Jack W. Davis; **Photographer (interior):** David P. Swain; **Art Manager:** Craig Newsom; **Illustrator:** Tom Roberts; **Printer:** United Graphics

Printed in the United States of America   10   9   8   7   6   5   4   3   2   1

Human Kinetics
Web site: www.humankinetics.com

United States: Human Kinetics, P.O. Box 5076, Champaign, IL 61825-5076
800-747-4457
e-mail: humank@hkusa.com

Canada: Human Kinetics, 475 Devonshire Road Unit 100, Windsor, ON N8Y 2L5
800-465-7301 (in Canada only)
e-mail: orders@hkcanada.com

Europe: Human Kinetics, Units C2/C3 Wira Business Park, West Park Ring Road, Leeds LS16 6EB, United Kingdom
+44 (0) 113 278 1708
e-mail: hk@hkeurope.com

Australia: Human Kinetics, 57A Price Avenue, Lower Mitcham, South Australia 5062
08 8277 1555
e-mail: liahka@senet.com.au

New Zealand: Human Kinetics, P.O. Box 105-231, Auckland Central
09-523-3462
e-mail: hkp@ihug.co.nz

Contents

Preface   vii

Acknowledgments   ix

Chapter 1 ▸ Case Studies and Risk Stratification   **1**

Screening and Risk Stratification   2
Assessing the Components of Fitness   10
Goal Setting   12
Exercise Prescription   14
References   14

Chapter 2 ▸ Basic Principles of Exercise Prescription, Now With $\dot{V}O_2$ Reserve   **15**

Principles of Training   15
ACSM Guidelines   21
$\dot{V}O_2$ Reserve   23
References   27

Chapter 3 ▸ Exercise Prescription for Cardiorespiratory Fitness   **29**

Type (Mode)   29
Frequency and Time (Duration)   30

Intensity   32

Exercise Prescription by Heart Rate   33

Exercise Prescription by Perceived Exertion   39

Exercise Prescription by Workload   41

References   42

Chapter 4▶ Using the ACSM Metabolic Equations   43

Functions of the Metabolic Equations   44

Conversion of Units   45

Walking   48

Running   51

Leg Cycling   55

Arm Cycling   58

Stepping   61

References   63

Chapter 5▶ Exercise Prescription for Weight Loss   65

Energy Balance   66

Weight Management   67

Exercise Prescription for Fat Loss   68

References   75

Chapter 6▶ Exercise Prescription for Muscular Strength and Flexibility   77

Flexibility   77

Muscular Strength   83

References   96

Chapter 7 ▶ Exercise Prescription for the Older Adult   97

Cardiovascular Fitness   98
Resistance Training   100
References   108

Chapter 8 ▶ Exercise Prescription for Heart Disease   111

Exercise for Heart Disease   112
Four Variables of the FITT Principle   112
Myocardial Infarction   114
Heart Failure   116
Pacemakers   117
Cardiac Transplant   119
References   121

Chapter 9 ▶ Exercise Prescription for Diabetes Mellitus   123

Exercise Prescription for
   Clients With Type 1 Diabetes   125
Exercise Prescription for
   Clients With Type 2 Diabetes   130
References   137

Chapter 10 ▶ Exercise Prescription for Other Special Cases   139

Peripheral Vascular Disease   139
Chronic Obstructive Pulmonary Disease   142
Hypertension   144
Pregnancy   146

Children   148

References   151

Appendix   Additional Case Studies With
Multiple Choice Questions   **153**

Index   181

About the Authors   189

Preface

Properly performed exercise has enormous health benefits. It reduces the risk of many diseases, increases functional capacity, and improves the quality of our lives. Simply choosing to be physically active on a daily basis will reap many of these benefits, but to truly optimize our health and fitness we need to integrate many facets of exercise into a well-designed program. The American College of Sports Medicine (ACSM) has taken a leading role in providing exercise professionals with the tools to design sound exercise prescriptions for clients ranging from the healthy to those with chronic diseases and from the young to the elderly. This book will help students and exercise professionals to put guidelines into practice. We explain the ACSM's recommendations for prescribing exercise and use numerous case studies to illustrate the key points. The case studies are realistic examples that provide a hands-on feel to exercise prescription. We believe you will find this book an invaluable aid in applying the science of exercise to your real-life clients.

The first chapter introduces the book's case study approach and then explains in detail how the ACSM stratifies clients into low-, moderate-, and high-risk groups. Such stratification is essential prior to designing exercise programs for clients. Chapter 2 provides an overview of the principles of exercise training, leading into the specifics of ACSM exercise prescriptions for cardiorespiratory fitness (chapter 3) and for muscular strength and flexibility (chapter 6). Chapter 4 teaches how to calculate the oxygen cost and energy expenditure of various forms of exercise—knowledge you will need in writing cardiorespiratory exercise prescriptions and in prescribing exercise for weight loss (chapter 5).

Chapters 7 through 10 apply the principles learned thus far to older adults (chapter 7), people with heart disease (chapter 8), people with diabetes mellitus (chapter 9), and other special populations such as pregnant women, children, and individuals with peripheral vascular disease, chronic obstructive pulmonary disease, or hypertension (chapter 10). We follow ACSM guidelines throughout the book, clearly delineating any instances where we as authors take issue with those recommendations. If you are using this text to study for ACSM certification at the Health / Fitness Instructor level, you should know that this certification does not cover clinical populations—yet any health fitness instructor should have a basic understanding of heart disease and diabetes, since these diseases are so widespread that you will often encounter such patients in the fitness setting.

Acknowledgments

We would like to thank Sheri Colberg, PhD, FACSM, for her constructive comments on the chapter concerning exercise and diabetes mellitus. Dr. Colberg is an Assistant Professor at Old Dominion University and author of the book *The Diabetic Athlete*.

1

Case Studies
and Risk Stratification

C ase studies are an excellent way to learn how to put knowledge into practice. Case studies provide the learning experience closest to dealing with real-life clients. In certification examinations, the American College of Sports Medicine uses case studies extensively to illustrate the principles of exercise prescription. The most popular ACSM certification, Health/Fitness Instructor, even devotes an entire station of the practicum exam to evaluating a case study.

The ACSM's approach to evaluating a case study involves three steps:

1. Screening and risk stratification
2. Assessment of the components of fitness
3. Exercise prescription

This chapter explores the ACSM's basic approach to evaluating case studies, with special attention to screening and risk stratification. Subsequent chapters of this book present case studies that emphasize different elements of this approach. The case studies in the appendix are comprehensive and challenge you to perform complete evaluations of a variety of real-life clients.

SCREENING AND RISK STRATIFICATION

Renowned exercise physiologist Per-Olaf Åstrand has often said that it is safer to exercise than to remain sedentary. This is almost universally true, because exercise produces many healthful benefits that reduce the risk of diseases associated with inactivity—coronary heart disease, cerebrovascular disease, type 2 diabetes, osteoporosis, certain forms of cancer, etc. Yet exercise carries some risk. It increases metabolic demands on the heart and increases sympathetic nervous activity—factors that could trigger a heart attack in individuals who already have coronary heart disease. Because the many people with undiagnosed heart disease are particularly at risk, screening clients is critical to insure safety. Before performing exercise testing on clients, and before enrolling them into an exercise program, you should evaluate the clients to determine their level of risk and to decide if it is reasonably safe to proceed.

ACSM's Risk Levels

- **Low-risk:** Young (less than 45 years old for men, less than 55 for women), with no more than one coronary disease risk factor, and without symptoms or known disease.

- **Moderate-risk:** Older (45 or more years for men, 55 or more for women); or with two or more coronary disease risk factors.

- **High-risk:** With one or more symptoms of cardiopulmonary disease; or with known cardiovascular, pulmonary, or metabolic disease. (Franklin 2000)

Table 1.1 provides a screening form for evaluating clients. The form lists all of the ACSM criteria for risk factor thresholds, symptoms, and relevant known diseases. Note that the ACSM screening criteria are intended specifically to determine a client's risk *prior to* exercise and are not intended as a complete list of coronary risk factors. For example, the ACSM is well aware of the fact that exposure to tobacco in any form—chewing tobacco, cigars, pipes, cigarettes, or second-hand smoke—elevates the risk of serious disease. Yet only active cigarette smoking appears on the screening list, in recognition of the greater risk from this form of exposure.

Table 1.1

Exercise Screening Questionnaire Using ACSM Criteria

Name _____ Sex _____ Date _____

I. Risk Factors (two or more places individual at moderate risk)

___ 1. Have any of your parents, brothers, or sisters had a heart attack, bypass surgery, angioplasty, or sudden death prior to the age of 55 (male relatives) or 65 (female relatives)?

___ 2. Have you smoked cigarettes in the past 6 months?

___ 3. What is your usual blood pressure ($\geq 140/90$)? Do you take blood pressure medication?

___ 4. What is your LDL cholesterol? If you don't know your LDL, what is your total cholesterol? What is your HDL cholesterol? [Either LDL > 130 (use total cholesterol > 200 if LDL not known) **OR** HDL < 35 is a risk. Note: HDL > 60 is a "negative" risk factor.]

___ 5. What is your fasting glucose (≥ 110)?

___ 6. What is your height and weight (BMI ≥ 30)? Also, what is your waist girth (> 100 cm)?

___ 7. Do you get at least 30 minutes of moderate physical activity most days of the week (or its equivalent)?

II. Symptoms (one or more places individual at high risk)

___ 1. Do you ever have pain or discomfort in your chest or surrounding areas? (i.e., ischemia)

___ 2. Do you ever feel faint or dizzy (other than when sitting up rapidly)?

___ 3. Do you find it difficult to breathe when you are lying down or sleeping?

___ 4. Do your ankles ever become swollen (other than after a long period of standing)?

___ 5. Do you ever have heart palpitations, or an unusual period of rapid heart rate?

___ 6. Do you ever experience pain in your legs (i.e., intermittent claudication)?

___ 7. Has a physician ever said you have a heart murmur? (Has he/she said it is OK, and safe for you to exercise?)

___ 8. Do you feel unusually fatigued or find it difficult to breathe with usual activities?

(continued)

Table 1.1   *(continued)*

III. Other

___ 1. How old are you? (Men ≥ 45, women ≥ 55 are at moderate risk.)

___ 2. Do you have any of the following diseases: heart disease, peripheral vascular disease, cerebrovascular disease, chronic obstructive pulmonary disease (emphysema or chronic bronchitis), asthma, interstitial lung disease, cystic fibrosis, diabetes mellitus, thyroid disorder, renal disease, or liver disease? (Yes to any disease places individual at high risk.)

___ 3. Do you have any bone or joint problems, such as arthritis or a past injury, that might get worse with exercise? (Exercise testing may need to be delayed or modified.)

___ 4. Do you have a cold or flu, or any other infection? (Exercise testing must be delayed.)

___ 5. Are you pregnant? (Exercise testing may need to be delayed or modified.)

___ 6. Do you have any other problem that might make it difficult for you to do strenuous exercise?

Interpretation

Low risk (young, and no more than 1 risk factor): can do maximal testing or enter a vigorous exercise program.

Moderate risk (older, or 2 or more risk factors): can do submaximal testing or enter a moderate exercise program.

High risk (one or more symptoms, or disease): can do no testing without physician presence; can enter no program without physician clearance.

Adapted, by permission, from *ACSM's Guidelines For Exercise Testing and Prescription,* 6th ed., 2000, edited by BA Franklin (Philadelphia: Lippincott Williams & Wilkins).

When screening clients, always explore the answers to their questions rather than taking simple answers at face value. For example, when asked "Do you ever have pain or discomfort in your chest or surrounding areas?" a client with a recent muscle strain during bench pressing would answer yes but would not be at elevated risk of heart disease. Coronary ischemia is not usually a sharp pain—rather, it appears as a pressure or discomfort, normally occurs during times of stress (including exercise), and is relieved by rest. Similarly, dizziness is common (and benign) when people sit up rapidly. Swelling of the ankles may not indicate cardiovascular complications if it results from long periods of standing with little movement. You must interpret clients' responses with prudent judgment—and, before continuing with exercise testing or programming, must refer to a physician any client whose symptoms might be due to cardiopulmonary disease.

The bottom of table 1.1 summarizes the ACSM's recommendations about the form of exercise testing and the intensity of exercise training that clients are ready to enter after the screening process. Low-risk clients are unlikely to experience cardiovascular complications during even the most strenuous exercise. Thus, you can offer low-risk clients submaximal or maximal exercise tests without a physician's supervision, and you can enter these clients into moderate or vigorous exercise programs without first obtaining a physician's clearance.

You can offer moderate-risk clients a submaximal exercise test, such as a bike test performed at a moderate intensity for the prediction of $\dot{V}O_2max$, but should not give them a maximal exercise test in a health club or other fitness site. Moderate-risk individuals should undergo maximal exercise testing only in a clinical setting (i.e., with a physician available in the immediate vicinity). They can enter moderate-intensity exercise programs such as walking clubs or moderate-intensity resistance training but not vigorous programs such as running or competitive sports. If they want to enter a vigorous exercise program, they must first obtain physician clearance—preferably involving a clinically supervised stress test.

High-risk clients should not receive any exercise testing or programming without the direct involvement of the medical community. Exercise tests should be medically supervised. Entry into any exercise program, even of a moderate intensity, needs to be preceded by physician clearance based on stress testing.

CASE STUDY 1.1
Risk Stratification

John S. is a 42-year-old who is 5'8" (173 cm) tall and weighs 178 lb (80.9 kg). He works as a construction laborer. He smokes about a pack of cigarettes per day, and has done so over 20 years. His father had a heart attack at age 61. John has no signs or symptoms of cardiopulmonary disease. His blood pressure is 136/82 mmHg

(continued)

Case Study 1.1 *(continued)*

on medication. His total cholesterol is 220 mg·dl⁻¹. His fasting glucose is 96 mg·dl⁻¹. He has come to your facility to learn more about ways to reduce his risk of heart disease. How many ACSM risk factors does he have, and what risk stratification category is he in? Can you perform a submaximal or maximal fitness test on him at this time? Can he enter a moderate or vigorous exercise program before obtaining physician clearance?

Mr. S. has three risk factors: cigarette smoking, hypertension (because he is on medication, even though his current blood pressure is reasonable), and hypercholesterolemia (based only on knowing his total cholesterol, which is above 200 mg·dl⁻¹). He is not obese, although his body mass index (BMI) of 27.1 kg·m⁻² puts him in the overweight category (table 1.2). He would not be classified as sedentary, due to his physically active job. He does not have a family history of heart disease *for screening purposes*, because his father's heart attack occurred after the age of 55. His fasting glucose is normal. Although Mr. S. is considered to be young (less than 45), he is in the moderate-risk category because he has at least two risk factors. He is not in the high-risk category, because he does not have any signs or symptoms of cardiopulmonary disease or any known cardiovascular, pulmonary, or metabolic disease.

Table 1.2

Body Mass Index Categories

BMI (kg·m⁻²)	Category	BMI (kg·m⁻²)	Category
<18.5	Underweight	30.0-34.9	Obesity, class I
18.5-24.9	Normal	35.0-39.9	Obesity, class II
25.0-29.9	Overweight	≥ 40.0	Obesity, class III (morbid)
≥ 30.0	ACSM criterion for obesity		

Note: BMI is calculated as body mass in kg divided by the square of height in meters. It may also be calculated from English units as follows: (body weight in lb × 703)/(height in inches squared). The factor 703 converts from English to metric units.

Adapted, by permission, from "Executive summary of the clinical guidelines on the identification, evaluation, and treatment of overweight and obesity in adults," *Archives of Internal Medicine* 158(17):1857. Copyright 1998 *American Medical Association.*

You can safely give Mr. S. a submaximal test of his cardiovascular fitness as part of an overall appraisal of his condition. He cannot undergo a maximal test unless physician coverage is available. Mr. S. can safely begin a moderate-intensity exercise program, but he would need physician clearance before embarking on a vigorous exercise program.

CASE STUDY 1.2
Risk Stratification

Joan D. is a 32-year-old sales consultant. She smoked three to five cigarettes per day until she quit nine months ago. She is 5'4" (163 cm) tall and weighs 128 lb (58.2 kg). Her grandfather died of heart disease when he was 63. Her mother has type 2 diabetes. Her blood pressure is 106/70 mmHg. She has a total cholesterol of 192 mg·dl^{-1}, LDL 134 mg·dl^{-1}, and HDL 46 mg·dl^{-1}; fasting glucose is 87 mg·dl^{-1}. She walks her dog for 15-20 minutes once or twice a day. Stratify Ms. D.'s risk status, and decide what type of exercise testing and programming she can perform.

Ms. D. has only one risk factor: hypercholesterolemia. Her total cholesterol is in the desirable range, but LDL cholesterol is more important than total cholesterol. Because her LDL is above the threshold level of 130 mg·dl^{-1}, she meets the criterion for this risk factor. Her HDL is normal, but *either* high LDL or low HDL levels place a client at risk. Ms. D. has been smoke-free for more than six months, so cigarette smoking is not a risk factor (risk for heart disease drops quickly after smoking cessation, approaching the risk of nonsmokers in one to two years; ex-smokers approach normal risk levels for lung cancer and pulmonary disorders in 10-20 years). Ms. D.'s BMI is normal at 22.0 kg·m^{-2}. The heart disease in Ms. D.'s grandfather and diabetes in her mother do not elevate her own risk of having a heart attack during exercise. Ms. D. would not be considered sedentary, because her three hours of walking per week exceeds the ACSM's recommendation of at least two hours of moderate activity per week (i.e., 30 minutes or more on most days of the week; if "most days" is interpreted to mean at least four out of seven, this yields a total of two hours or more per week).

(continued)

Case Study 1.2   *(continued)*

Because Ms. D. has only one risk factor and is young (less than 55 years old), she is in the low-risk category. You can give her a maximal test of her aerobic capacity without a physician present. However, you may not need a maximal test: a submaximal test would provide sufficient information to proceed with her exercise prescription. Ms. D. can safely enter a moderate or a vigorous exercise program. If you prescribe a vigorous exercise program, be sure to set the initial intensity at a level appropriate for her current level of fitness—not out of fear of a heart attack, but to prevent excessive musculoskeletal strain at the onset of her program.

CASE STUDY 1.3
Risk Stratification

Andy B. is a 58-year-old public school teacher who is 5'11" (180 cm) tall and weighs 188 lb (85.5 kg). He is a nonsmoker, with blood pressure of 136/94 mmHg. His brother recently underwent bypass surgery at the age of 52. He plays an hour or more of tennis several afternoons a week and walks 18 holes of golf on Sundays. He complains of pain in the elbow of his dominant arm and of soreness in his ankles. He has no other signs, symptoms, or chronic diseases. His lipid profile is 187 mg·dl^{-1}, 106 mg·dl^{-1} for LDL, and 68 mg·dl^{-1} for HDL; fasting glucose is 96 mg·dl^{-1}. Stratify Mr. B.'s risk status, and decide what type of exercise testing and programming he can perform.

Mr. B. has two risk factors: hypertension and family history. But because his HDL cholesterol is favorably high (above 60 mg·dl^{-1}), subtract one risk factor. For screening purposes he therefore has only one risk factor, which would put him in the low-risk category if he were younger. However, because he is at least 45 years old, he is automatically placed in the moderate-risk category. Note that hypertension is a risk factor, even though only one of the two blood pressure readings, the diastolic in his case, is high. His BMI of 26.2 kg·m^{-2} is slightly overweight, but it does not meet the criterion for obesity. His frequent exercise keeps him out of the sedentary category and is the most likely cause of his orthopedic complaints. You can give Mr. B. a submaximal exercise test and prescribe a moderate exercise program at your facility without the need for physician clearance.

CASE STUDY 1.4
Risk Stratification

Alana K. is a 62-year-old executive in your corporation. During a wellness fair that you provided, the following information was gathered. She is a nonsmoker. She is 5'6" (168 cm) tall, weighs 224 lb (101.8 kg), and has a waist girth of 43" (109 cm). Her blood pressure is 128/84 mmHg, and her lipid profile is: total cholesterol of 218 mg·dl^{-1}, LDL cholesterol of 141 mg·dl^{-1}, HDL cholesterol of 52 mg·dl^{-1}. Fasting glucose is 122 mg·dl^{-1}. Her father died of a heart attack at age 74, and her mother and one of her sisters have type 2 diabetes. Her main form of recreation is reading. She reports no signs or symptoms of chronic diseases. Stratify Ms. K.'s risk status, and decide what type of exercise testing and programming she can perform.

Ms. K. has three risk factors: obesity, hypercholesterolemia, and impaired fasting glucose. Obesity is met by two separate criteria—a BMI over 30 kg·m^{-2} (hers is 36.2 kg·m^{-2}) and a waist circumference over 100 cm. Hypercholesterolemia is determined because her LDL reading was over 130 mg·dl^{-1}. Her fasting glucose is well above the cutoff of 110 mg·dl^{-1}. Note that the fasting glucose test should be repeated to be certain that it is *typically* this high. A fasting glucose >126 mg·dl^{-1} is the criterion for diagnosing diabetes, but only a physician can make a diagnosis. In a wellness fair, you can only tell her that her fasting glucose is high and that she needs to follow up with her physician.

Technically speaking, Ms. K. is in the moderate-risk category. You can offer her submaximal testing and moderate-intensity exercise programming. However, it would be prudent to wait for her physician's judgment regarding her impaired fasting glucose (i.e., borderline diabetes) before beginning her program.

CASE STUDY 1.5
Risk Stratification

Walter R. is a 21-year-old college student. He is a varsity track athlete, competing in the shot put and hammer throw. He is 6'1" (185 cm) tall and weighs 245 lb (111 kg). His measured body fat is 14%. He is a nonsmoker, and his blood pressure is 128/84 mmHg.

(continued)

Case Study 1.5 *(continued)*

His father passed away from a sudden cardiac event at the age of 42. No blood cholesterol or glucose data are available. Mr. R. complains of dizziness when he has to run wind sprints with the track team, and he once passed out briefly after practice. He is being assessed as part of a college wellness class. Stratify his risk.

At first glance, Mr. R. has two risk factors: obesity and family history. Obesity is based on his BMI (32.3 kg·m⁻²) being above the criterion of 30 kg·m⁻². However, because he is a strength athlete, his high BMI may be due simply to his large musculature. This is confirmed by his low body fat measurement, thus he would not be considered obese. More troubling than his risk factors is his complaint of dizziness and syncope during high-intensity exercise. This symptom raises a red flag and automatically places Mr. K. in the high-risk category. He may have a serious congenital abnormality of the heart (which his father may also have had), and it is essential that he be referred to a physician. In fact, you should tell him not to participate in any exercise until he is clinically evaluated.

ASSESSING THE COMPONENTS OF FITNESS

After you screen and stratify clients, your next step is usually to assess their fitness in various areas. Fitness assessment is not mandatory before entering a client into an exercise program, but it is a highly useful step that gives you baseline information to help you design your exercise prescription. It is also useful to repeat assessments at regular intervals to evaluate the client's progress and modify the program. The ACSM emphasizes five components of fitness that have great relevance to health and to functional independence:

1. Body composition (% fat versus % lean body mass; but may also be judged from waist circumference or body mass index)
2. Aerobic capacity (maximal aerobic power, $\dot{V}O_2$max)
3. Muscular strength (maximal muscular force, 1-RM)
4. Muscular endurance (ability to repeat a given level of contractile force for multiple repetitions)
5. Flexibility (range of motion at a given joint)

You also may want to consider other components of fitness, particularly if athletic performance is at issue. Such additional components would include, but not be limited to, the following: aerobic endurance, lactate and/or ventilatory thresholds, anaerobic power, anaerobic capacity, reaction time, and balance.

Population norms for the five health-related components of fitness are presented in chapter 4 of the *ACSM's Guidelines for Exercise Testing and Prescription,* 6th edition. The ACSM considers the 90th percentile to be "well above average," the 70th percentile "above average," the 50th percentile "average," the 30th percentile "below average," and the 10th percentile "well below average" (Franklin 2000). These tables will serve as the basis of the fitness interpretations of subsequent case studies, but it is important to recognize that population norms have certain limitations.

One limitation is the population specificity of normative tables. The groups that were tested to provide the norms may not be representative of the types of clients at your facility. For example, some of the ACSM norms are from data collected by the Cooper Institute for Aerobics Research in Dallas. This institution has tested large numbers of clients, thus providing a measure of validity to these norms, but the clients who are able to afford testing at this prestigious institute are hardly representative of average Americans.

Another limitation of norms is that they indicate only what subjects in the test population *were able* to do, not what they *should be able* to do. For example, the average (50th percentile) push-up score for women in their 40s is listed as 12 modified (knees on floor) push-ups, whereas the "above average" (70th percentile) score is listed as 18 modified push-ups. Does this mean that 18 modified push-ups by a 40-something woman is laudatory? Does this truly reflect a high level of muscular fitness, or does it simply reflect low ability in the test group? Because norms are derived from the largely sedentary general population, they may not provide a realistic view of attainable fitness levels, especially in the older cohorts.

A different way to interpret a client's fitness is to employ **criterion standards**—i.e., levels of ability you feel are achievable or desirable—rather than **normative standards.** Our suggestion is that you use population norms (such as those provided by the ACSM) only as a starting point in working with clients, tailoring goals to clients' individual abilities and needs.

GOAL SETTING

The most important consideration in setting goals is that **the client must set the goals.** You may have a wealth of information about the client, such as body composition data, fitness test scores, lipid values, etc.; and you have the knowledge and experience to know what would be healthful and prudent goals for a given client. But if you simply inform your clients of their new goals during a consultation, they may not take them to heart. It is important for you to lead your clients into discovering the goals they should set for themselves. Always maintain a positive and encouraging attitude that helps your clients understand what would be appropriate goals; and be sufficiently open-minded to see when clients are not interested in the goals you feel are appropriate.

Lay out the current situation to the client: "Your aerobic capacity is such-and-such, which for your age and sex is a little below average. More importantly, it places you at a higher risk for heart disease and means that you can't enjoy many recreational activities." Suggest what would be appropriate and attainable goals: "Fortunately, you can make some real progress in this area with the right exercise program. If you put the effort into it, we could help you to reach the above-average category in just a few months. That would significantly reduce your risk of heart disease and give you the capacity to enjoy an afternoon of tennis without feeling exhausted afterwards. On the other hand, a more modest program would at least allow you to reach the average category and help you to maintain a reasonable level of fitness for the coming years." Ask the client to set the goal: "What would you like to accomplish? Where would you like to be a year from now?"

Some other important factors to consider in goal setting:

1. Goals should be challenging but attainable.
2. Help clients to set long-term and short-term goals.
3. Goals should be highly specific and practical.
4. Enlist social support to help clients reach their goals.

Goals should be challenging but attainable. Don't fall into the pattern of expecting little progress from a client, because in your experience many clients don't make dramatic improvements. Dramatic improvements are indeed possible, and you need to project confidence that the client can make great changes. Ask clients to think about how they would really like to be a year or two from now. Lose 100 pounds and look fit and trim? Lower total cholesterol from 300 to well under 200 mg·dl^{-1}? Improve aerobic capacity from couch potato status to marathon finisher? All of these are very achievable for most people, and you should give clients the motivation to reach for their dreams. However, changes like these do not happen overnight: "I've never run before and I want to run a marathon next month." "Great, but let's aim for next year." And some goals may be unrealistic: "I want to be national champion in my sport someday." "You've been competing in your sport for several years and are still at a regional level; we can help you improve, but your aerobic power/ muscle strength/whatever isn't likely to reach elite levels."

Lofty goals for the future are admirable, provided they are also realistic, but what will the client accomplish in the next week or month? Help clients break down long-term goals into short-term, manageable segments. This provides a framework for setting workout plans and evaluating progress. It also provides frequent reinforcement as clients attain intermediate goals. A desire to lose 100 pounds in the next two years can be lost if the individual sees no progress in the next two weeks.

Goals to improve fitness, lower cholesterol, or lose weight are appropriate as a starting point. But such general goals are not meaningful in a practical sense. Goals must be translated into a highly specific, personalized plan of action. Consider a goal to lower cholesterol by 50 points through a decrease in dietary fat intake. To what specific new food choices is the client committing? Drinking skim milk instead of whole, eating fish instead of red meat, using olive oil instead of saturated and hydrogenated fats? The client needs goals associated with adopting new behaviors, not just numbers from a blood test. Or consider a goal to improve aerobic capacity from the average to the above average category. This goal needs to be expressed in terms of behavior change, in association with a detailed exercise prescription. For example, the client may commit to walking briskly for 20-30 minutes four times a week. When, exactly, will she do this walking? Ask her to verbalize the days of the week and the times of day when she will walk. Write it down as part of the exercise prescription. Of course, some flexibility is needed in putting these changes into action, but obtaining a clear commitment from the client *for specific behaviors,* and not just outcomes, makes the goal more concrete and more likely to be accomplished.

Social support is a key element to successful behavior change. Humans are social animals, and much of human behavior is based on seeking the approval of others. If family members or coworkers scoff at clients' new behaviors, it will be much harder for them to achieve their goals. Try to turn clients' desire for approval to their advantage: involve family members in the program; run team contests at work sites; enlist partners in a buddy system; target highly visible and respected people for programming, such as company CEOs. Tapping into the power of social support is an important ingredient in helping clients to achieve their goals.

EXERCISE PRESCRIPTION

The exercise prescription is the next step after clients are screened and their goals established; yet writing exercise prescriptions and establishing goals are interrelated tasks. It is not practical to design a fully developed exercise prescription without knowing a client's goals, but some basic principles of exercise prescription apply to most situations. Chapter 2 discusses these principles; and table 2.1 summarizes the associated ACSM guidelines.

To be certified as an ACSM Health/Fitness Instructor, one must be able to verbalize and apply these general guidelines. To work with clients in day-to-day practical situations, you should be able to master the details of these guidelines to set specific exercise prescriptions that are tailored to the needs of individual clients. Subsequent chapters will explore these guidelines for exercise prescription in more detail.

REFERENCES

1. Expert Panel. 1998. Executive summary of the clinical guidelines on the identification, evaluation, and treatment of overweight and obesity in adults. *Arch. Int. Med.* 158:1855-1867.

2. Franklin, BA, ed. 2000. *ACSM's Guidelines for Exercise Testing and Prescription*, 6th ed., 24-27. Philadelphia: Lippincott Williams & Wilkins.

2

Basic Principles of Exercise Prescription, Now With $\dot{V}O_2$ Reserve

The principles for prescribing exercise have been developed over centuries of human activity and athletic conditioning and refined over the past few decades of scientific research. This chapter presents an overview of these principles and introduces the American College of Sports Medicine guidelines for exercise prescription that will be followed throughout this book.

PRINCIPLES OF TRAINING

Living organisms adapt to stress. This basic aspect of all life is the foundation of exercise training. If individuals increase their effort a little more than normal (called an "overload" by exercise physiologists), their bodies will respond by improving strength or flexibility or aerobic capacity or any other component of fitness that the activity challenged. Although any form of overload induces a response, to get the best results one needs to perform the exercise in a well-designed, systematic fashion.

Years of research have uncovered several guiding principles for optimum exercise training. Of special note are the principles of overload, adaptation, progression, specificity, recovery, overtraining, detraining, and individual responsiveness.

Overload and Adaptation

In figure 2.1, the vertical axis presents the maximum capacity of a system. This capacity could refer to aerobic power (i.e., maximal oxygen consumption, $\dot{V}O_2max$), to muscular strength (i.e., one repetition maximum, 1-RM), or to some other capacity. Each bout of exercise—when performed as an **overload**—initially results in fatigue and a temporary decrease in capacity. As the system recovers from the bout of exercise, the capacity increases to a level greater than the original value (figure 2.1a). This increase is due to a number of physiological **adaptations** that are inherent to living things.

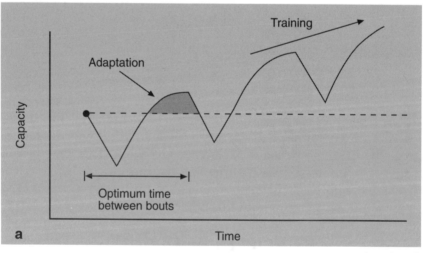

(continued)

Figure 2.1 Illustration of the adaptive response of training. (*a*) The proper spacing of exercise bouts allows full recovery and adaptation, resulting in *training*. (*b*) Bouts are spaced too close together, preventing full recovery and resulting in *overtraining*. (*c*) Bouts are spaced too far apart, resulting in a loss of adaptation and *detraining*.

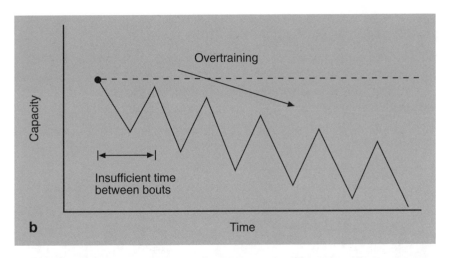

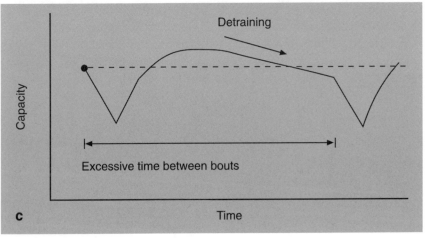

Figure 2.1 *(continued)*

For a partial list of these adaptations, see "Adaptations to Aerobic Training" on page 18 and "Adaptations to Resistance Training" on page 19. Most of these changes are typically too small to be measured after a single bout of exercise, but their cumulative effect over many bouts of exercise is referred to as training.

Progression

The principle of **progression** states that *the exercise stimulus must increase over time in order to elicit continued improvements.* For example,

Adaptations to Aerobic Training

- Increased parasympathetic tone/decreased sympathetic tone—reduced HR at rest and during submaximal exercise, slightly reduced maximal HR
- Increased size of the left ventricle (proportional increase in wall thickness and chamber diameter, eccentric hypertrophy)—increased stroke volume at rest and during both submaximal and maximal exercise
- Increased cardiac output, workload, and oxygen consumption at maximal exercise
- Increased plasma volume
- Increased maximal ventilation, decreased ventilation during submaximal exercise (improved economy of breathing)
- Decreased resistance to blood flow in trained muscles—reduced BP at rest and during submaximal exercise
- Increased number of capillaries—reduced diffusion distance for oxygen
- Increased myoglobin in muscle cells—increased oxygen transport to mitochondria
- Substantial increase in mitochondria and associated enzymes
- Increased use of fat—glycogen-sparing, increased endurance at submaximal workload
- Increased insulin sensitivity
- Increased lactate removal by organs—increased lactate threshold, tolerance of high intensity effort
- Increased ATP, CP, and glycogen stores

lifting a 10-lb dumbbell in a biceps curl might increase a person's strength; but if that person stays with that weight for several weeks, the strength will increase only in the first week or two but will not improve after that point. The intensity or the duration or the frequency of the stimulus must gradually increase for gains in strength to continue. A popular variation of this principle is periodization, in which the stimulus varies in a structured pattern over time, including periods of relative recovery—yet the overall effect is that the stimulus increases.

Adaptations to Resistance Training

▶ Increased motor unit recruitment—ability to simultaneously contract a greater percentage of motor units

▶ Increased growth of myofilaments—muscle cell hypertrophy, and thus muscle hypertrophy

▶ Possible long-term conversion of type 1 to type 2 fibers

▶ Possible proliferation of muscle cells (hyperplasia)—muscle hypertrophy

▶ Increased stores of ATP, CP, and glycogen

▶ Increased left ventricle size (wall thickness more than chamber diameter, concentric hypertrophy)

Specificity

It is important to recognize that the adaptations induced by training are highly **specific** to the stress. One obvious example is that resistance training increases strength but has a minimal effect on aerobic capacity. Furthermore, the increased strength arises in the muscles that were exercised but not in other muscles (although a small amount of crossover improvement can be observed in the muscles of the opposite limb when only one limb is trained, due to neural adaptations). These examples are obvious, but they illustrate a principle that is present in more subtle applications. An example: resistance training on an isokinetic machine (which varies the resistance to produce a constant angular speed of movement at a joint) results in large increases in strength *on that device.* But when the isokinetically trained muscles perform similar movements using standard machines or free weights (that have a constant external load), they will exhibit much smaller increases in strength. The reason for this effect is that *most of the strength increase after resistance training is due to improved **neural recruitment patterns,*** which are specific to the way in which the muscle is asked to contract. Only a small portion of the strength improvement is due to muscle hypertrophy, which is generalized to any activity performed by the muscle. An example of specificity from aerobic training is that very little of the improvement in aerobic capacity after one mode of training (e.g., running) is evident when the individual performs a different mode of exercise that uses many of the same muscle groups (e.g., cycling).

Recovery, Overtraining, Detraining

In figure 2.1, the horizontal axis presents time, and the distance between bouts of exercise is the **recovery** time. Workouts must be spaced carefully to obtain the best results. The body needs time to recover and replenish energy stores and for adaptive processes to take place. The length of recovery time needed between bouts varies directly with the overall stress (both the intensity and volume) of the exercise session. Obviously, highly intense or lengthy bouts of exercise require greater recovery times than less intense or shorter bouts. If the bouts are spaced too closely together, insufficient recovery will take place before the next session occurs, leading to **overtraining** (figure 2.1b); if too much time occurs between bouts, the adaptation will be lost and **detraining** will occur (figure 2.1c).

The optimum spacing of workouts depends on numerous interdependent factors, chief among them being the overall stress of the workout; the type of exercise being performed (e.g., resistive, aerobic, flexibility); and the person's current training status, fitness level, and nutritional status. People typically perform resistance training only once every two or three days, but the schedule varies with the intensity of the workout. During rehabilitation from an injury, resistance training may occur as often as twice per day but with very low resistance. Alternatively, some weightlifting athletes may train a given muscle group as infrequently as once a week, to provide sufficient recovery from extremely intense exercise. Aerobic training is generally performed at least three times per week but can be done daily or even twice daily in both rehabilitation and athletic conditioning. Endurance athletes must build up to such high training frequency (and duration) over an extended period of time, and they must pay special attention to nutritional needs (primarily, a high carbohydrate intake to replenish glycogen stores), to orthopedic tolerance, and to signs of overtraining. Flexibility training is best done on a daily or twice-daily basis, but less frequent training can still yield meaningful results.

Individual Responsiveness

The adaptive responses of the human body to various exercise regimens are well known and allow exercise professionals to develop exercise prescriptions and workout routines that can be widely applied to the general population. However, individual responses to training will vary. Some clients improve more quickly than others.

As discussed earlier, recovery time between workouts can vary considerably due to many individual factors. Furthermore, many clients may have orthopedic conditions or health problems, or may be taking a variety of medications, that require special consideration in exercise prescription. For these reasons, you must consider national guidelines, such as those of the American College of Sports Medicine, as a starting point in working with clients. Always be prepared to adjust workloads up or down based on the immediate responses of a client to an exercise session, as well as on the overall progress that the client is making over time.

ACSM GUIDELINES

The American College of Sports Medicine has taken a leading role in the study of exercise physiology and the practice of exercise prescription. Its recommendations have been published since the first edition of *Guidelines for Graded Exercise Testing and Exercise Prescription* in 1975 (ACSM 1975), and they have been systematically reviewed and refined in succeeding editions. In 1998, the ACSM published a landmark position stand in its scientific journal, *Medicine and Science in Sports and Exercise,* on "The Recommended Quantity and Quality of Exercise for Developing and Maintaining Cardiorespiratory and Muscular Fitness, and Flexibility in Healthy Adults" (Pollock et al. 1998). This position stand synthesized a vast body of knowledge about the scientific aspects of exercise training and put forth recommendations for exercise prescription. In 2000, these recommendations were further presented in the sixth edition of *ACSM's Guidelines for Exercise Testing and Prescription* (Franklin 2000), the "bible" of exercise professionals.

Table 2.1 summarizes the ACSM's current recommendations for aerobic training, resistance training, and flexibility training. These recommendations are intended to provide a framework for exercise professionals who work with the general population, as opposed to the opposite extremes of patients or athletes. However, as later chapters will explore, the basic principles require only modest modifications when working with these specialized groups. These guidelines follow the *FITT* principle, where *F* stands for frequency of exercise (days per week), *I* for intensity (% of maximum capacity), *T* for time (duration on a given day) and *T* for type (the mode of exercise).

The term "HRR" in tables 2.1 and 2.2 refers to **heart rate reserve**— i.e., a percentage of the difference between resting and maximal HR.

Table 2.1

ACSM Exercise Prescription Principles

Category	Frequency	Intensity	Time	Type
Cardiovascular	3-5 days per week	40/50-85% of HRR or $\dot{V}O_2R$	20-60 minutes	Large muscle mass, continuous, rhythmic
Muscular strength	2-3 days per week	8-12 RM range	1 set each of 8-10 exercises ($\leq$ 1 hr)	Major muscle groups, full ROM, controlled speed
Flexibility	2-3+ days per week	To mild discomfort	10-30 sec for each of 3-4 reps	Static or assisted (PNF)

Adapted, by permission, from *ACSM's Guidelines For Exercise Testing and Prescription,* 6th ed., 2000, edited by BA Franklin (Philadelphia: Lippincott Williams & Wilkins), 73.

Table 2.2

Equivalent Exercise Intensities Using %HRR, %$\dot{V}O_2R$, and %$\dot{V}O_2$max

%HRR	%$\dot{V}O_2R$	%$\dot{V}O_2$max		
		5-MET capacity	10-MET capacity	20-MET capacity
0% (rest)	0%	20%	10%	5%
40%	40%	52%	46%	43%
50%	50%	60%	55%	53%
85%	85%	88%	87%	86%
100%	100%	100%	100%	100%

%HRR units and %$\dot{V}O_2R$ units provide equivalent intensities throughout the range from rest to maximal exercise—e.g., if a client is at 50% of heart rate reserve, he or she is also at 50% of $\dot{V}O_2$ reserve. Units of %$\dot{V}O_2$max must be adjusted to achieve the same intensity. Furthermore, the amount of adjustment needed in the %$\dot{V}O_2$max units varies with the fitness level of the client. The table illustrates this principle for three different clients, one with a 5-MET capacity (deconditioned), one with a 10-MET capacity (average sedentary adult), and one with a 20-MET capacity (endurance athlete).

The term "$\dot{V}O_2R$" refers to $\dot{V}O_2$ **reserve,** which is similarly defined as a percentage of the difference between resting and maximal $\dot{V}O_2$. Intensity for resistance training is indicated as "8-12 RM," which means the range from the 8-repetition maximum to the 12-repetition maximum. The 8-RM is a weight that can be lifted 8 times in succession but not 9 times. Such a weight is approximately 84% of a person's 1-RM. Similarly, a 12-RM load is a weight that can be lifted 12 but not 13 times and is approximately 76% of 1-RM. The term "ROM" means **range of motion.** Under flexibility training, the term "PNF" refers to **proprioceptive neuromuscular facilitation.** This is a mode of stretching in which the client actively contracts a muscle against resistance (often supplied by the trainer), followed by relaxation of the muscle while it is stretched. The specific information presented in table 2.1 will be examined in much more detail in the succeeding chapters and applied to a variety of practical case studies.

$\dot{V}O_2$ RESERVE

The introduction of $\dot{V}O_2$ reserve is an important change made by the ACSM in its 1998 position stand and 2000 *Guidelines*. Previously, the ACSM recommended that exercise prescriptions for cardio-respiratory fitness be based on a percentage of $\dot{V}O_2$max. It had been assumed that clients could be placed at a given percentage of $\dot{V}O_2$max by having them exercise at that same percentage of heart rate reserve. That is, if one wished a client to exercise at 60% of $\dot{V}O_2$max, the target HR would be calculated at 60% of HRR (take 60% of the difference between HRmax – HRrest, and then add this product to HRrest).

However, recent research demonstrated that there is an error between %HRR and %$\dot{V}O_2$max (Swain and Leutholtz 1997, 1998). This error is easiest to observe at rest. When a person is resting, he or she is by definition at 0% of HRR (0% of a *range* is simply the low end of the range) but is not at 0% of $\dot{V}O_2$max, since that would be a $\dot{V}O_2$ of 0. The person would have to be dead, not resting, to be at 0% of $\dot{V}O_2$max! As figure 2.2 shows, the error between %HRR and %$\dot{V}O_2$max *at rest* can be quite large, depending on the client's fitness level. A typical person has a $\dot{V}O_2$ at rest of 3.5 ml·min^{-1}·kg^{-1} (or 1 MET) and a $\dot{V}O_2$max that is 10 times higher, or 35 ml·min^{-1}·kg^{-1} (i.e., 10 METs). This person would therefore be at 1/10 of $\dot{V}O_2$max, or 10%, when resting. A poorly fit client, with a maximal capacity of only 17.5 ml·min⁻¹·kg⁻¹, or 5 METs, would be at 1/5, or 20% of $\dot{V}O_2$max at rest. On the other hand, there is very little error between %HRR and %$\dot{V}O_2$max for highly fit clients, as illustrated in figure 2.2 by the individual with a 20-MET capacity (70 ml·min⁻¹·kg⁻¹) who is at 1/20, or 5%, of $\dot{V}O_2$max when resting.

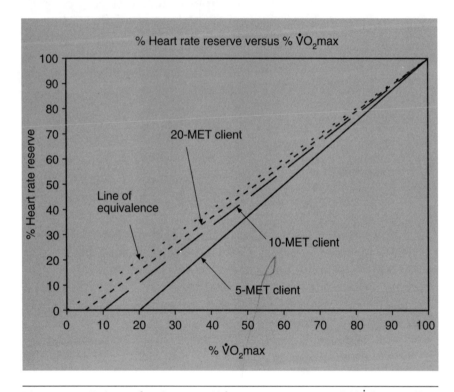

Figure 2.2 Relationship between % heart rate reserve and %$\dot{V}O_2$max, illustrating a large discrepancy between these two indicators of intensity, especially at lower levels of exercise (i.e., the distance between the solid lines and the line of identity). This discrepancy between %HRR units and %$\dot{V}O_2$max units is larger for clients with lower fitness levels, as seen by the greater distance from the line of identity for the 5-MET client compared to the 10-MET and 20-MET clients.

The error between %HRR and %$\dot{V}O_2$max becomes gradually smaller as exercise intensity increases, since both %HRR and %$\dot{V}O_2$max are approaching 100%. The error is most noticeable in clients with a low fitness level, exercising at a low intensity. In research by the current authors, we introduced the term "$\dot{V}O_2$ reserve" to rep-

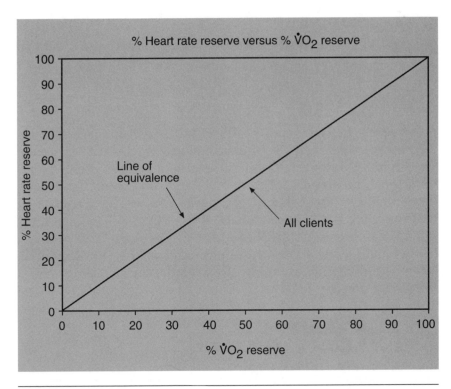

Figure 2.3 In contrast to figure 2.2, the relationship between %HRR and %$\dot{V}O_2$ reserve falls along the line of identity (i.e., %HRR units and %$\dot{V}O_2$R units provide equivalent indicators of exercise intensity). This is true for clients of all fitness levels, making %$\dot{V}O_2$R very useful for exercise prescription.

resent the percentage of the difference between resting and maximal $\dot{V}O_2$. Of course, when a person is resting, he or she is at 0% of HRR and also 0% of $\dot{V}O_2$R. Consequently, we demonstrated that there is no error between these terms throughout the range of exercise intensities, from rest up to maximum (figure 2.3). That is to say, a client can be placed at any desired percentage of $\dot{V}O_2$R by using that same percentage of HRR: 40% of HRR is equivalent to 40% of $\dot{V}O_2$R, 60% of HRR is equivalent to 60% of $\dot{V}O_2$R, and so on. Table 2.2 provides the values of %HRR, %$\dot{V}O_2$R, and %$\dot{V}O_2$max at equivalent levels of exercise intensity. Values of %$\dot{V}O_2$max are presented for three individuals with different fitness levels. Fitness level does not affect the values for %HRR and %$\dot{V}O_2$R, as all clients are placed at similar levels of intensity *relative to their own ability* by using these terms. Use the following formula to calculate a target intensity using $\dot{V}O_2$R:

$\dot{V}O_2$ Reserve Formula:

Target $\dot{V}O_2$ = (intensity fraction)($\dot{V}O_2$max – $\dot{V}O_2$rest) + $\dot{V}O_2$rest

Since resting $\dot{V}O_2$ averages 3.5 ml·min^{-1}·kg^{-1}, this can be rewritten as

Target $\dot{V}O_2$ = (intensity fraction)($\dot{V}O_2$max – 3.5) + 3.5

Our research used young, healthy adults exercising on both cycle ergometers and treadmills. After its publication, the ACSM adopted the use of $\dot{V}O_2$R for establishing intensity in exercise prescriptions in its position stand (Pollock et al. 1998) and in its Guidelines (Franklin 2000). Since that time, other researchers have confirmed that an error exists between %HRR and %$\dot{V}O_2$max—and that there is a no error between %HRR and %$\dot{V}O_2$R—in older, healthy adults (Down and Haennel 1997) and in cardiac patients (Brawner et al. 2000). The following case study illustrates the effect of using %$\dot{V}O_2$R in exercise prescriptions.

CASE STUDY 2.1

Use of %$\dot{V}O_2$R vs. %$\dot{V}O_2$max in an Exercise Prescription

Susan H. is a 57-year-old woman who is very deconditioned. She is 5'5" tall (165 cm) and weighs 187 lb (85 kg). Her body mass index (BMI) is 31 kg·m^{-2}, which places her in the class I obesity category. She is sedentary, has a family history of heart disease, and has an elevated resting blood pressure (146/92 mmHg). Because she recently complained of shortness of breath, her physician ordered a stress test. She performed the modified Bruce protocol and completed stage I (1.7 mph, 10% grade) with a maximal HR of 158 bpm and no indications of coronary ischemia. Her aerobic capacity was estimated from the treadmill protocol as 5 METs (i.e., 17.5 ml·min^{-1}·kg^{-1}). What is an appropriate exercise prescription to improve her aerobic conditioning?

At this point we will not examine a detailed treatment of Ms. H.'s current condition and exercise prescription—only the issue of how the use of %$\dot{V}O_2$R versus %$\dot{V}O_2$max affects the prescription. Due to her poor fitness status, you should set her initial exercise intensity at a low level. According to table 2.1, the ACSM recommends that a prescription can begin as low as 40% of $\dot{V}O_2$R. You decide that her target $\dot{V}O_2$ during exercise will be as follows:

$$\text{Target } \dot{V}O_2 = (\text{intensity fraction})(\dot{V}O_2\text{max} - 3.5) + 3.5$$
$$= 0.40(17.5 - 3.5) + 3.5$$
$$= 0.40(14) + 3.5$$
$$= 5.6 + 3.5$$
$$= 9.1 \text{ ml·min}^{-1}\text{·kg}^{-1}$$

As chapter 4 will explain, the ACSM's metabolic equations can translate a target $\dot{V}O_2$ into a workload on a piece of exercise equipment. In this case, 9.1 ml·min^{-1}·kg^{-1} yields a treadmill walking speed of 2.1 mph. If 40% of $\dot{V}O_2$max had been used instead of 40% of $\dot{V}O_2$R, the target $\dot{V}O_2$ would have been only $0.40 \times 17.5 = 7$ ml·min^{-1}·kg^{-1}, which translates to a walking speed of 1.3 mph. Thus, the use of %$\dot{V}O_2$max would have placed her at a walking speed that is almost 40% less than she actually needs. Furthermore, if you use a target HR to determine her exercise intensity, you need to recognize that 40% of HRR would result in the higher of these two walking speeds.

In case study 2.1, %$\dot{V}O_2$max introduced a large error in the prescribed exercise intensity, relative to the client's ability. As mentioned earlier, the error would be smaller for more fit clients or for clients exercising at higher percentages of their capacity. The use of %$\dot{V}O_2$max in exercise prescriptions for endurance athletes introduces only minimal errors. Nevertheless, for the sake of consistency, this book will follow the ACSM's recommendation of using %$\dot{V}O_2$R instead of %$\dot{V}O_2$max whenever there is a need to establish an exercise intensity from $\dot{V}O_2$.

REFERENCES

1. ACSM. 1975. *Guidelines for Graded Exercise Testing and Exercise Prescription.* Philadelphia: Lea & Febiger.

2. Brawner, CA, LN Gibson, JK Ehrman, and SJ Ketayian. 2000. Percent heart rate reserve is equivalent to percent $\dot{V}O_2$ reserve among patients with myocardial infarction (abstract). *Med. Sci. Sports Exerc.* 32(Suppl.):S142.

3. Down, RJ, and RG Haennel. 1997. Percent heart rate reserve is not equivalent to percent maximal oxygen uptake (abstract). *Can. J. Appl. Physiol.* 22(Suppl.):13P.

4. Franklin, BA, ed. 2000. *ACSM's Guidelines for Exercise Testing and Prescription*, 6th ed., 137-164. Philadelphia: Lippincott Williams & Wilkins.

5. Pollock, ML, GA Gaesser, JD Butcher, JP Despres, RK Dishman, BA Franklin, and CE Garber. 1998. The recommended quantity and quality of exercise for developing and maintaining cardiorespiratory and muscular fitness, and flexibility in healthy adults (ACSM Position Stand). *Med. Sci. Sports Exerc.* 30:975-991.

6. Swain, DP, and BC Leutholtz. 1997. Heart rate reserve is equivalent to $\%\dot{V}O_2$Reserve, not to $\%\dot{V}O_2$max. *Med. Sci. Sports Exerc.* 29:410-414.

7. Swain, DP, BC Leutholtz, ME King, LA Haas, and JD Branch. 1998. Relationship of % heart rate reserve and $\%\dot{V}O_2$Reserve in treadmill exercise. *Med. Sci. Sports Exerc.* 30:318-321.

3

Exercise Prescription for Cardiorespiratory Fitness

As noted in chapter 2 and summarized in table 2.1, cardiorespiratory exercise prescriptions are based on the *FITT* principle: Frequency, Intensity, Time (duration), and Type (mode). This chapter briefly examines type, frequency, and time, and then explains in detail the ACSM's recommendations for prescribing intensity.

TYPE (MODE)

A cardiorespiratory exercise is one that stimulates a substantial, sustained increase in oxygen consumption. To do this, the exercise must utilize a large amount of muscle mass. Thus, while operating a rowing machine with just the arms is aerobic, it is not as effective for cardiorespiratory training as performing the exercise with the arms, legs, and back. To obtain a sustained increase in oxygen consumption, the exercise must be continuous and rhythmic: repetitive activities like walking, running, rowing, bicycling, and swimming are more aerobic than stop-and-go sports like tennis and basketball.

FREQUENCY AND TIME (DURATION)

The recommended frequency of cardiorespiratory exercise is three to five days per week, with a duration of 20 to 60 minutes per day (Franklin 2000). Most clients just starting an exercise program are able to begin with three times a week for 20 minutes. Depending on their goals, they should then progress toward the upper range of frequency and duration (possibly increasing intensity as well). Progression should occur gradually and be tailored to individual responsiveness to the training program. A prudent goal for many clients would be to increase the total volume of exercise by 10% per week.

The exercise time can be accumulated over two or more sessions in a day to achieve the desired total, although one cannot simply add up various daily chores and term this a training program. Sixty one-minute trips to the water fountain do not add up to an hour of aerobic exercise! Each exercise session needs to be a distinct period of time in which the proper intensity is maintained, not including the warm-up and warm-down.

Both warm-ups and warm-downs should entail 5-10 minutes of low-intensity exercise that emphasizes the same muscles used in the exercise session. The warm-up period increases the temperature and elasticity of the muscles and elicits increases in breathing, heart action, and muscle blood flow that prepare the body for the more vigorous exercise to come. The warm-down prevents blood pooling by maintaining the "muscle pump" effect in which the active muscles massage their own veins to help propel blood toward the heart. The warm-down also helps clear lactic acid from the bloodstream.

Flexibility training is best done at the end of the warm-down when the muscles are still warm and elastic. Clients who like to do stretching before they exercise should be instructed to delay the stretching at least until after they have completed their warm-up.

A frequency of less than three days per week may not be sufficient for improving cardiorespiratory fitness, although it may allow for maintenance of a moderate fitness level. A frequency greater than five days per week will provide diminishing returns of improvement for the amount of time and effort expended, and it may lead to overtraining or orthopedic problems. Yet most people, if they increase their schedule quite gradually, can successfully perform cardiorespiratory exercise on a daily basis. People who exercise three or four times per week should to do so on alternate days, to allow their bodies maximum recovery time between sessions.

The ACSM recommends that the duration of 20 to 60 minutes should be used in a complementary manner with intensity. To burn a given number of calories, or to achieve a desired amount of overload, people can exercise at a high intensity for a short period of time, or at a low intensity for a long period of time. In practice, most fit clients exercise with a longer duration *and* a higher intensity than less fit clients; but the ACSM recommendations aim to develop a desirable level of health-related fitness for the general population.

CASE STUDY 3.1

Cardiorespiratory Exercise Prescription

Yolanda L. is a 33-year-old, moderate-risk client. She is overweight and sedentary but otherwise appears healthy. She states that she would like to become more fit, but she has trouble finding time in her schedule for exercise. Design a general exercise program for her to improve cardiorespiratory fitness.

Ask Ms. L. if there are any types of aerobic exercise that she enjoyed when she was younger, or enjoys watching other people perform. Help her select a mode of exercise that is fun and that entails little initial equipment or expense. For many clients, walking is a great choice. If she tries one mode of exercise for a couple of weeks and doesn't like it, help her to choose another. Explain to her that exercise is critical to health, and that she should make an initial commitment to perform 20 minutes of exercise, three times a week, at a moderate intensity. (The initial intensity should be 50% of $\dot{V}O_2R$; prescribing intensity will be explained in more detail later in this chapter.) Help her to find a specific time, or times, in her day when she is doing things that are of lower priority. (To make time for exercise, many people might choose to watch less television in the evenings, or go to bed a little earlier and then exercise in the morning, or schedule an exercise break during the workday, etc. Without health, all other pursuits in life are unattainable. Thus, most activities earn a lower priority than regular exercise.) Be sure also to teach Ms. L. how to warm up and warm-down.

Next, discuss exercise progression with her. Although she is starting with 20 minutes, three times a week, she will want to gradually increase her exercise duration to achieve the best results. For example, each week she could add five minutes to each

(continued)

Case Study 3.1 *(continued)*

exercise session, until she reaches perhaps an hour. She could divide the hour into two or three sessions per day if that helps her achieve her duration goal. And she could add one day every other week, until she is working out five days per week. And she could increase the intensity gradually so that she feels the workout remains challenging while still being enjoyable (not to exceed the ACSM upper limit of 85% $\dot{V}O_2R$). You can reevaluate her in one or two months, and every few months thereafter, adjusting the program to best meet her goals. Once she reaches her goals, help her set new ones—or enjoy a maintenance program that has no further increases in the exercise but might replace some of the exercise sessions with other recreational activities.

INTENSITY

Intensity of exercise should be based on oxygen consumption. Both the oxygen delivery system and the oxygen consumption of the muscles must be challenged with an overload. This is why the recommended intensity is set at a percentage of aerobic capacity and specifically at a percentage of $\dot{V}O_2$ reserve. Of course, unless people are exercising in a laboratory, direct knowledge of their oxygen consumption is not available—and so you must translate the percentage of $\dot{V}O_2$ reserve into a term that your client can use. There are three ways to do this:

Ways to Prescribe the Intensity of Aerobic Exercise

1. Exercise prescription by heart rate
2. Exercise prescription by perceived exertion
3. Exercise prescription by workload

Regardless of the method you use, it should result in a range of intensity that falls between 50% and 85% of $\dot{V}O_2$ reserve (Franklin 2000). The ACSM notes that the minimum intensity of 50% can be reduced to as low as 40% and still provide some benefit to individuals who start with a very low fitness level. A recent analysis suggests that the minimum intensities should be lowered from 50% to 45% $\dot{V}O_2$ reserve for moderately to highly fit clients and from 40% to 30% of $\dot{V}O_2$ reserve for clients with a low fitness level (Swain and

Franklin, in press). However, because this recommendation has not yet been incorporated into the ACSM's position stands, this book will follow the current ACSM guidelines. Generally, individual clients should be prescribed an intensity range that is narrower than the overall range of 40/50% to 85% of VO_2 reserve. For example, you might prescribe 50-60% for someone who is just beginning an exercise program, but you would prescribe 70-80% for a more fit client.

Why doesn't the ACSM recommend the use of higher intensities, from 85-100% of VO_2 reserve? Certainly, high intensities are very effective at increasing VO_2max, especially when used in intervals, such as several repetitions of three to five minutes at 95-100% alternated with three to five minutes of active recovery. The ACSM recommendations are intended not for athletes but for members of the general population who wish to improve fitness and reduce their risk of disease. Intensities approaching 100% effort may result in burnout for many people and also carry greater risk of injury or cardiovascular complications.

EXERCISE PRESCRIPTION BY HEART RATE

Heart rate varies in a very linear manner with oxygen consumption during aerobic exercise. If a certain increase in oxygen demand results in a 10 bpm increase in heart rate, then twice that demand for oxygen will increase heart rate by 20 bpm. This linear response is very useful because you can measure a client's heart rate very easily by palpation or by relatively inexpensive monitors. Further, because heart rate provides a good reflection of oxygen consumption, you can use it as a surrogate for oxygen consumption in writing exercise prescriptions. Remember that you are interested in the change in oxygen consumption, not the change in heart rate. A heart rate that is elevated for several minutes during a scary movie does *not* provide an aerobic training effect! Similarly, an elevated pulse during anaerobic exercise, such as weightlifting, does not indicate an aerobic effect.

There are two popular ways to prescribe exercise intensity by heart rate: the percentage of maximal heart rate method (%HRmax) and the percentage of heart rate reserve method (%HRR).

Percent HRmax Method

This is a simple way to calculate a target heart rate, although its exclusion of resting HR limits its usefulness to some degree. The formula for the %HRmax method is simple:

> Target Heart Rate by %HRmax Method:
>
> Target HR = (intensity fraction)(HRmax)

Choose the intensity fraction to provide the appropriate intensities of $\dot{V}O_2$ reserve. It is important to recognize that the same numerical values for %HRmax and for %$\dot{V}O_2$R give different exercise intensities. To achieve a desired level of %$\dot{V}O_2$R, you must use a higher value for the %HRmax number. According to the ACSM's sixth edition *Guidelines*, 55% HRmax corresponds to 40% $\dot{V}O_2$R, 65% HRmax to 50% $\dot{V}O_2$R, and 90% HRmax to 85% $\dot{V}O_2$R (Franklin 2000). *However, these %HRmax values are too low according to available research* (Londeree and Ames 1976; Swain et al. 1994). These values have recently been revised upward (Howley, in press); table 3.1 provides the appropriate values of %HRmax for different levels of %$\dot{V}O_2$R.

Table 3.1

Equivalent Exercise Intensities of %$\dot{V}O_2$R, %HRR, %HRmax, and RPE for Prescribing Exercise

%$\dot{V}O_2$R	%HRR	%HRmax*	RPE
40%	40%	64%	12
50%	50%	71%	13
60%	60%	77%	14
70%	70%	84%	15
80%	80%	91%	16
85%	85%	94%	17

Cardiorespiratory exercise intensity may be prescribed as a workload (based on a desired percentage of $\dot{V}O_2$ reserve), as a target heart rate (calculated by the %HRR method or the %HRmax method), or as a rating of perceived exertion. Percent HRR units provide equivalent intensities to %$\dot{V}O_2$R units, while %HRmax units must be adjusted upwards to provide the same intensities. (* Equivalent values for %HRmax are from Howley, in press.)

You will rarely know the true maximal heart rates of clients, but you can obtain a reasonable estimate by subtracting an individual's age in years from 220 bpm. Note, however, that this is only an estimate—approximately two-thirds of the population will have maximal heart rates that are within 10 bpm of the calculated figure (220 – age); thus, one-third will have maximal heart rates that are more than 10 bpm higher or lower than the estimate, and about 5% of normal subjects will have maximal heart rates more than 20 bpm from the estimate. For this reason, *it is much better to use a true maximal heart rate if it is available.* Although such tests are rarely performed outside a clinical environment, one can determine maximal heart rate by having a subject exercise to exhaustion in a graded exercise test.

If you do estimate maximal heart rate as 220 – age (or use other available formulas), remember that the target HR is also just an estimate. Use the target HR as a starting point, and be prepared to adjust the exercise intensity based on the client's response. After you have worked with the client, it would be appropriate to modify the target HR values based on your professional judgment.

CASE STUDY 3.2
Exercise Prescription Using %HRmax

Tawana R. is a 37-year-old woman who wishes to enter your aerobic dance class. She has already been screened and is in the low-risk category. During the class, you will be starting with a warm-up and gradually building to a fairly vigorous routine. You tell the class participants to check their HR frequently to see that they are working within the target zone. Using the %HRmax method, what are Ms. R.'s upper and lower limits of the HR range? If you use a 10-second count in your class, what number of beats should she be looking for?

Because Ms. R. is low-risk, she can exercise anywhere within the 50-85% $\dot{V}O_2R$ range. She should reach or exceed the 50% level by the end of the class warm-up and should use the 85% level as an upper limit for the vigorous sections of the class. Based on table 3.1, her target HRs would be set at 71-94% of maximum. Her maximal HR is estimated as 220 – 37 = 183 bpm.

$$\text{Lower target HR} = (0.71)(183)$$
$$= 130 \text{ bpm}$$
$$\text{Upper target HR} = (0.94)(183)$$
$$= 172 \text{ bpm}$$

To express these targets as 10-second counts, divide the HRs in bpm by 6, yielding a range of 22-29 beats.

CASE STUDY 3.3
Exercise Prescription Using %HRmax

Pedro S. is a 24-year-old, low-risk client. He runs recreationally for three miles, 4-5 times per week. He finds it very difficult to maintain an even pace, especially when going up and down hills. After screening, you perform a fitness evaluation and find that his $\dot{V}O_2$max is approximately 44 ml·min^{-1}·kg^{-1}. You encourage him to purchase a heart rate monitor, using it to maintain a steady intensity rather than a steady speed. Using the %HRmax method, what HR range would you recommend to him?

Mr. S. has an aerobic capacity that is slightly above average (at the 60th percentile, based on chapter 4 of the ACSM sixth edition *Guidelines*). You could choose any intensity between 50-85% of $\dot{V}O_2$R, but it would be reasonable to narrow that down to 60-70% in light of his current fitness status. After he has practiced for a week with his HR monitor, you can adjust the intensity range depending on his response. According to table 3.1, the corresponding target HR range is 77-84% of HRmax. His estimated HRmax is $220 - 24 = 196$ bpm.

$$\text{Lower target HR} = (0.77)(196)$$
$$= 151 \text{ bpm}$$
$$\text{Upper target HR} = (0.84)(196)$$
$$= 165 \text{ bpm}$$

Because the %HRmax method of prescribing exercise intensity is so simple to use, it is very popular. Unfortunately, it is limited because it does not account for resting HR. Consider an exercise prescription for a 70-year-old woman with a resting HR of 90 bpm. If you placed her at the lowest intensity, 64% of HRmax (i.e., 40% of $\dot{V}O_2$R), the target HR would be $(0.64)(220 - 70) = 96$ bpm. The target HR is barely more than her resting HR!

Or consider an exercise prescription for two 30-year-olds, one of whom has a resting HR of 50 bpm and the other of 80 bpm. If you place both at an intensity of 71% of HRmax (i.e., 50% of $\dot{V}O_2$R), you would give both a target HR of $(0.71)(220 - 30) = 135$ bpm. However, this is an increase of 85 bpm above rest for the first client and an increase of only 55 bpm above rest for the second. Clearly, these two clients would not be exercising at the same intensity. The client with the lower resting heart rate would have a much higher relative intensity.

The **heart rate reserve method** avoids the problems associated with variations in resting HR.

Percent HRR Method

Heart rate reserve is simply the difference between resting and maximal heart rate. Because Karvonen et al. (1957) first used a percentage of this range to establish exercise intensity, this method is often called the **Karvonen method.** As chapter 2 explains, subsequent research has shown that %HRR provides intensities of exercise equivalent to the values of %$\dot{V}O_2$ reserve. Regardless of a person's age or fitness level or resting heart rate, the HRR method provides accurate target heart rates relative to desired percentages of $\dot{V}O_2$ reserve.

The formula for calculating a target HR by the %HRR method is as follows:

Target Heart Rate by %HRR Method:

Target HR = (intensity fraction)(HRmax – HRrest) + HRrest

The intensity fraction is the same numerical value as the desired percentage of $\dot{V}O_2R$. As with the %HRmax method, you can estimate maximal HR by subtracting age from 220; but always use a client's actual maximal HR if you know it. Optimally, you should measure resting HR after several (at least five) minutes of quiet rest. If the client is agitated, or has just been engaged in stressful activity, the measured HR will not reflect true resting conditions. The quiet rest is best performed in a seated position, especially if the client's main form of exercise is bicycling, rowing, or some other seated activity. If the client's main form of exercise is performed in an upright posture (e.g., walking, running), it would be appropriate to have the client stand for two to three minutes after the seated rest period and then to measure the HR.

CASE STUDY 3.4
Exercise Prescription Using %HRR

Jeremy C. is a 64-year-old, moderate-risk client. He wants to begin an exercise program to reduce his risk of heart disease. His

(continued)

Case Study 3.4 *(continued)*

physician has performed a stress test to evaluate his condition, and there are no indications of clinically relevant heart disease at this time. His measured maximal HR is 148 bpm, with resting HR of 86 bpm. Using the %HRR method, what would be an appropriate target HR range?

You place Mr. C. at the low end of the normal intensity range, 50-60% of $\dot{V}O_2R$, and therefore 50-60% of HRR. You could estimate his maximal HR as $220 - 64 = 156$ bpm, but you instead use the known value of 148 bpm. You prescribe his target HR range as follows:

$$\text{Lower target HR} = (0.50)(148 - 86) + 86$$

(Remember basic laws of algebra: first perform functions that are within parentheses, then perform multiplications or divisions, then perform additions or subtractions.)

$$= (0.50)(62) + 86$$
$$= 31 + 86$$
$$= 117 \text{ bpm}$$
$$\text{Upper target HR} = (0.60)(148 - 86) + 86$$
$$= (0.60)(62) + 86$$
$$= 37 + 86$$
$$= 123 \text{ bpm}$$

Note that, if instead you had used the %HRmax method, you would have obtained the following target HRs, based on a lower limit of 71% HRmax (for 50% $\dot{V}O_2R$) and an upper limit of 77% HRmax (for 60% $\dot{V}O_2R$):

$$\text{Lower target HR} = (0.71)(148)$$
$$= 105 \text{ bpm}$$
$$\text{Upper target HR} = (0.77)(148)$$
$$= 114 \text{ bpm}$$

With a large number of clients, *average* target HRs should be similar with both %HRmax and %HRR methods. In Mr. C.'s case, however, the %HRmax values come out too low. The %HRR method is slightly more cumbersome mathematically, but it provides a more individually tailored prescription—therefore it is the preferred method of prescribing HR in most settings.

EXERCISE PRESCRIPTION BY PERCEIVED EXERTION

Heart rate is an excellent measure for prescribing exercise intensity, but it's not for everyone. Many people can gauge the intensity of their exercise by how hard it feels. Athletes have been doing this for generations, although the use of HR monitors has recently become quite popular in certain sports. Other individuals may wish to use HR but may not be able to do so because of clinical conditions (such as autonomic neuropathy) or medications (such as beta-blockers) that impair the HR response to exercise. (Individuals on beta-blockers can still use HR, provided their exercise prescription is based on HR data collected while on the medication.) Some medications (including such readily available drugs as caffeine and nicotine) may elevate rather than impair heart rate, making the heart rate prescription inaccurate.

Other conditions can also influence heart rate. For example, exercising in the heat elevates the heart rate above what would otherwise be expected, and pregnancy reduces the range of heart rates available to the exercising woman (resting HR is increased and maximal HR is reduced). Finally, some individuals simply find it too difficult to measure their own heart rate.

One way of prescribing exercise that relies on an individual's own perception of effort is the **talk test.** If a client is still able to talk during an exercise session—i.e., can speak in complete sentences without gasping for breath—then the intensity is not excessive. Of course, this provides only an upper limit; you can describe the lower limit to a client as being "hard enough to make you aware that you are breathing harder."

The talk test effectively places most clients in an aerobic training zone, but exercise scientists have sought to quantify perceived exertion with numerical scales that provide a reasonable correlation to exercise intensity. The most popular such scale is the **Rating of Perceived Exertion (RPE) scale** designed by Borg (1982). The scale, which ranges from 6 to 20, is intended to correspond to heart rates of 60 to 200 bpm in young adults. Individuals of any age can use the scale, with 6 representing rest and 20 maximal effort. Descriptors (such as "very light" and "somewhat hard") are provided for each odd number on the scale. Ask clients to use the numbers or descriptors as a reflection of their *overall feeling of effort* when exercising, not just how tired their legs feel or how hard they are breathing.

The ACSM cautions that RPE scales are subjective and should be carefully compared with actual exercise intensity *on an individual basis*. However, the ACSM does provide approximate equivalencies between the Borg scale and percentages of $\%\dot{V}O_2R$ (Franklin 2000). Table 3.1 lists these equivalencies. As with any variable used to prescribe the intensity of exercise, use the RPE only as a starting point; be prepared to adjust the intensity based on the client's responses. For example, one client might report an RPE of 15 during a given exercise, yet visibly appear to be exerting very little effort. If the prescription calls for a "hard" intensity, it would be appropriate to increase the workload gradually and ask the client to reevaluate how "hard" the exercise really is.

CASE STUDY 3.5

Exercise Prescription Using RPE and %HRR

Sarah P. is a 42-year-old, moderate-risk client. She has a resting HR of 68 bpm. You want her to exercise at an intensity equivalent to 50-70% of $\dot{V}O_2R$. She finds manual measurement of HR to be difficult but says that she might purchase a HR monitor. What would be her target HR using the %HRR method, and what would be an equivalent intensity range based on the Borg RPE scale?

You estimate Ms. P.'s maximal HR as $220 - 42 = 178$ bpm. According to table 3.1, the RPE values that correspond to 50-70% $\dot{V}O_2R$ are 13-15, or "somewhat hard" to "hard." This range should correspond to the following target HRs:

$$\text{Lower target HR} = (0.50)(178 - 68) + 68$$
$$= (0.50)(110) + 68$$
$$= 55 + 68$$
$$= 123 \text{ bpm}$$
$$\text{Upper target HR} = (0.70)(178 - 68) + 68$$
$$= (0.70)(110) + 68$$
$$= 77 + 68$$
$$= 145 \text{ bpm}$$

EXERCISE PRESCRIPTION BY WORKLOAD

The third way of prescribing exercise intensity, in addition to heart rate and perceived exertion, is by workload. What would be an appropriate speed and grade on a treadmill, or resistance setting and cadence on a cycle ergometer, or wattage on a stair stepper or rowing machine? If you can tell your clients how intense the setting should be on a piece of equipment, or how fast they should be walking or jogging outdoors, then they can be at the proper exercise intensity without having to use heart rate. For clients who cannot use heart rate, exercise prescription by workload provides a more objective way to set intensity than does RPE.

Exercise scientists have performed many studies to quantify the oxygen consumption during different types of exercise. Some modes of exercise have highly predictable oxygen demands, whereas others are much more variable.

The *predictable modes of exercise* are those in which the workload is easily measured and for which the exerciser is able to maintain a steady intensity over time—walking, running, and stationary cycling. For these modes of exercise, equations have been developed that allow you to estimate the oxygen consumption with reasonable accuracy regardless of the age, sex, weight, or skill level of the exerciser (chapter 4 will discuss these equations in detail). Armed with this information, you can provide clients with appropriate workload intensities in exercise prescriptions.

The *variable forms of exercise* are those in which skill greatly affects efficiency (e.g., swimming) or in which the intensity varies throughout an exercise session. Whereas the intensity of swimming is certainly related to the speed of movement through the water, the level of skill exhibited by individual swimmers has an enormous impact on the oxygen demand, making it impossible to provide a single equation that describes the oxygen demand with accuracy.

Other examples of exercises with variable intensity are tennis, basketball, and soccer. Although people can certainly obtain a good workout through these activities, the intensity of the exercise depends on the pace of a particular game, how much effort the individual chooses to use, and how much the opponent chooses to use! Tables have been compiled that provide general ranges of the oxygen consumption, or **MET** levels, for these activities (Ainsworth et al. 2000). Remember that *one MET is the average oxygen consumption at rest, 3.5 ml·min^{-1}·kg^{-1}*. Thus, the MET level is the oxygen consumption expressed as multiples of resting metabolism. It is possible to use these MET tables to assign intensity in an exercise prescription. However, because individuals choose to use quite variable levels of effort, the potential ranges of intensity in such activities are much greater than even the tables indicate—making prescription by this method of limited value. You can make accurate intensity prescriptions only for the highly predictable modes of aerobic exercise. Chapter 4 will introduce the mathematical equations used to quantify the workload in such cases.

REFERENCES

1. Ainsworth, BE, WL Haskell, MC Whitt, ML Irwin, AM Swartz, SJ Strath, WL O'Brien, DR Bassett, KH Schmitz, PO Emplaincourt, DR Jacobs, and AS Leon. 2000. Compendium of physical activities: an update of activity codes and MET intensities. *Med. Sci. Sports Exerc.* 32(9 suppl):S498-504.

2. Borg, G. 1982. Psychophysical bases of perceived exertion. *Med. Sci. Sports Exerc.* 14:377-381.

3. Franklin, BA, ed. 2000. *ACSM's Guidelines for Exercise Testing and Prescription*, 6th ed., 145, 150. Philadelphia: Lippincott Williams & Wilkins.

4. Howley, ET. In press. Type of activity: resistance, aerobic, anaerobic and leisure-time versus occupational physical activity. *Med. Sci. Sports Exerc.*

5. Karvonen, MJ, E Kentala, and O Mustala. 1957. The effects of training on heart rate: a longitudinal study. *Ann. Med. Exp. Biol. Fenn.* 35:307-315.

6. Londeree, BR, and SA Ames. 1976. Trend analysis of the %$\dot{V}O_2$max-HR regression. *Med. Sci. Sports Exerc.* 8:122-125.

7. Swain, DP, KS Abernathy, CS Smith, SJ Lee, and SA Bunn. 1994. Target heart rates for the development of cardiorespiratory fitness. *Med. Sci. Sports Exerc.* 26:112-116.

8. Swain, DP, and BA Franklin. In press. $\dot{V}O_2$ Reserve and the minimal intensity for improving cardiorespiratory fitness. *Med. Sci. Sports Exerc.*

4

Using the ACSM Metabolic Equations

The ACSM has developed equations for estimating oxygen consumption during walking, running, stationary cycling, and stepping (Franklin 2000). The equations are reasonably accurate for a wide range of individuals, because neither age, sex, nor skill strongly affects the energy demands of these modes of exercise. Body size does affect the energy demands, but this is accounted for in the equations.

The ACSM equations are fairly accurate, but they are only estimates. Therefore workload prescriptions or weight loss calculations based on these equations are estimates as well. As with prescriptions that use heart rate or perceived exertion to establish intensity, always observe a client's responses to the prescribed workload and be prepared to make adjustments.

The ACSM's equations are modified every few years, as new research warrants. The equations published in the 6th edition of the ACSM's *Guidelines* (Franklin 2000) have been significantly revised from those in previous editions: A term for unloaded cycling (the oxygen cost of moving the legs themselves) has been added to the leg cycling equation; a term for resting metabolism has been added to the stepping equation; and all equations have been formatted to yield answers for oxygen consumption in the units ml·min⁻¹·kg⁻¹ (Swain 2000). This book uses the equations that appear in the ACSM's 6th edition, summarized in table 4.1.

Table 4.1

The ACSM's Metabolic Equations

Walking

$\dot{V}O_2 = 3.5 + 0.1(\text{speed}) + 1.8(\text{speed})(\text{fractional grade})$

Running

$\dot{V}O_2 = 3.5 + 0.2(\text{speed}) + 0.9(\text{speed})(\text{fractional grade})$

Leg cycling

$\dot{V}O_2 = 7 + 1.8(\text{work rate})/(\text{body mass})$

Arm cycling

$\dot{V}O_2 = 3.5 + 3(\text{work rate})/(\text{body mass})$

Stepping

$\dot{V}O_2 = 3.5 + 0.2(\text{stepping rate}) + 2.4(\text{stepping rate})(\text{step height})$

Where:

$\dot{V}O_2$ is ml·min⁻¹·kg⁻¹

Speed is in m·min⁻¹

Work rate is in kg·m·min⁻¹

Body mass is in kg

Stepping rate is in steps per min

Step height is in m

Adapted, by permission, from *ACSM's Guidelines For Exercise Testing and Prescription*, 6th ed., 2000, edited by BA Franklin (Philadelphia: Lippincott Williams & Wilkins), 303.

FUNCTIONS OF THE METABOLIC EQUATIONS

You can use the metabolic equations for two purposes. **First, use them to calculate the oxygen consumption, and thus the energy expenditure, of a specific exercise.** This is valuable when you want to determine how many calories a client is burning during an exercise session and how much weight loss can be anticipated. **Second, you can use the equations to calculate the target workload in an exercise prescription.** In cases where heart rate or RPE may not be preferred, you can tell your client the intensity of exercise as a specific workload on a piece of exercise equipment or as a walking or running speed outdoors.

The metabolic equations yield oxygen consumption in gross terms. That is, they provide an individual's *total* oxygen consumption, including both the $\dot{V}O_2$ needed for resting metabolism and the additional $\dot{V}O_2$ needed for the exercise itself. To determine the *net* $\dot{V}O_2$, for example, when determining the number of calories that an exercise session expends above rest, simply subtract $3.5 \ ml \cdot min^{-1} \cdot kg^{-1}$ from the gross value.

$$\text{Gross } \dot{V}O_2 = \text{resting } \dot{V}O_2 + \text{exercise } \dot{V}O_2$$
$$\text{Gross } \dot{V}O_2 = 3.5 \ ml \cdot min^{-1} \cdot kg^{-1} + \text{net } \dot{V}O_2$$
$$\text{net } \dot{V}O_2 = \text{gross } \dot{V}O_2 - 3.5 \ ml \cdot min^{-1} \cdot kg^{-1}$$

CONVERSION OF UNITS

Depending on the situation, some of the terms used in the ACSM metabolic equations may not be in appropriate units. For example, rather than having oxygen consumption in the units $ml \cdot min^{-1} \cdot kg^{-1}$, one might need to express it in $L \cdot min^{-1}$, or in METs, or even in $kcal \cdot min^{-1}$ of energy expenditure. Likewise, you may need to alter the units for workload in the various equations. For example, speed is indicated in $m \cdot min^{-1}$, but you might prefer mph or kph. And cycling workload is in $kg \cdot m \cdot min^{-1}$ (which is not technically power), while you may prefer a measurement using watts. Table 4.2 provides the factors for converting between these various units.

Here is the simplest approach to using the equations:

1. Convert any raw data into the units as they appear in the equations.

2. Solve the equation using basic algebra.

3. If necessary, convert the answer into desired units.

This approach is followed in case studies later in this chapter.

Table 4.2

Conversion Factors for Metabolic Equations

$$\frac{(\dot{V}O_2 \text{ in L·min}^{-1}) \times 1000}{\text{body mass}} = \dot{V}O_2 \text{ in ml·min}^{-1}\cdot\text{kg}^{-1}$$

$$\frac{(\dot{V}O_2 \text{ in ml·min}^{-1}\cdot\text{kg}^{-1})(\text{body mass})}{1000} = \dot{V}O_2 \text{ in L·min}^{-1}$$

$$(\dot{V}O_2 \text{ in METs}) \times 3.5 = \dot{V}O_2 \text{ in ml·min}^{-1}\cdot\text{kg}^{-1}$$

$$\frac{(\dot{V}O_2 \text{ in ml·min}^{-1}\cdot\text{kg}^{-1})}{3.5} = \dot{V}O_2 \text{ in METs}$$

$$(\dot{V}O_2 \text{ in L·min}^{-1}) \times 5 = \text{energy exp. in kcal·min}^{-1}$$

$$\frac{\text{energy exp. in kcal·min}^{-1}}{5} = \dot{V}O_2 \text{ in L·min}^{-1}$$

$$(\text{speed in mph}) \times 26.8 = \text{speed in m·min}^{-1}$$

$$\frac{\text{speed in m·min}^{-1}}{26.8} = \text{speed in mph}$$

$$\frac{\text{speed in kph}}{0.06} = \text{speed in m·min}^{-1}$$

$$(\text{speed in m·min}^{-1}) \times 0.06 = \text{speed in kph}$$

$$\frac{\text{work rate in kg·m·min}^{-1}}{6} = \text{power in W}$$

$$(\text{power in W}) \times 6 = \text{work rate in kg·m·min}^{-1}$$

(Note: kg·m·min^{-1} is not technically a unit of power; also, conversion with the acceleration of gravity yields a correction factor of 6.12 . . . ; however, the ACSM uses 6 as a reasonable approximation for exercise prescriptions.)

$$\frac{\text{weight in lb}}{2.2} = \text{mass in kg}$$

$$(\text{mass in kg}) \times 2.2 = \text{weight in lb}$$

(Note: pounds are not a unit of mass, but can be converted with the factor 2.2 when the mass in question is subject to earth's gravity; for greater precision, a factor of 2.2046 can be used.)

$$\frac{\text{height in m}}{0.0254} = \text{height in inches}$$

$$(\text{height in inches}) \times 0.0254 = \text{height in m}$$

WALKING

The energy cost of walking increases in direct proportion with speed over the normal range of walking speeds. When a person tries to walk *extremely* fast, the energy cost increases exponentially. Thus, the walking equation should be used only for normal walking speeds, not race walking. The equation is accurate for treadmill or overground walking. When walking on flat ground (i.e., the grade is zero), the last term in the equation drops out. The equation has not been validated for walking downhill.

CASE STUDY 4.1

Walking—Solve for the $\dot{V}O_2$

George W. is a 51-year-old, moderate-risk client who weighs 163 lb. Due to his high-stress job, he has recently started an exercise program in the company wellness facility. He has selected his treadmill workload at a comfortable level, which is walking at 3 mph up a 6% grade. What is his estimated gross oxygen consumption in $ml \cdot min^{-1} \cdot kg^{-1}$, and what is the net number of calories he is burning each minute?

The first step is to convert any terms into the units requested by the equations. Thus, convert speed in mph to $m \cdot min^{-1}$, and weight in lb to mass in kg. Select the appropriate conversion factors from table 4.2.

$$3 \text{ mph} \times 26.8 = 80.4 \text{ } m \cdot min^{-1}$$
$$163 \text{ lb}/2.2 = 74.1 \text{ kg}$$

Second, select the walking equation from the list in table 4.1, enter all of the known variables, and solve for the unknown $\dot{V}O_2$. Remember to enter the grade as a fraction (0.06), not in percent units.

$$\dot{V}O_2 = 3.5 + 0.1(\text{speed}) + 1.8(\text{speed})(\text{fractional grade})$$
$$= 3.5 + 0.1(80.4) + 1.8(80.4)(0.06)$$

(In solving algebraic equations, always perform multiplications or divisions before doing additions or subtractions.)

$$= 3.5 + 8.04 + 8.6832$$
$$= 20.2 \text{ } ml \cdot min^{-1} \cdot kg^{-1}$$

Mr. W. is exercising with a gross $\dot{V}O_2$ of a little more than 20 ml·min^{-1}·kg^{-1}. To determine his net caloric expenditure, first subtract resting oxygen consumption from the gross value:

$$\text{Net } \dot{V}O_2 = 20.2 - 3.5 = 16.7 \text{ ml·min}^{-1}\text{·kg}^{-1}$$

If you had wanted net $\dot{V}O_2$ at the outset, you could simply have dropped the 3.5 from the walking equation when you first solved the problem.

Third, convert this oxygen consumption to a caloric expenditure. As seen in table 4.2, there is no direct conversion between ml·min^{-1}·kg^{-1} and kcal·min^{-1}. But there is an intermediate term, L·min^{-1}, that can serve as a bridge between the two.

$$\frac{16.7 \text{ ml·min}^{-1}\text{·kg}^{-1} \times 74.1 \text{ kg}}{1000} = 1.237 \text{ L·min}^{-1}$$

$$1.237 \text{ L·min}^{-1} \times 5 \text{ kcal·L}^{-1} = 6.2 \text{ kcal·min}^{-1}$$

During his treadmill walking, Mr. W. is burning approximately 6.2 kcal·min^{-1} above his resting energy expenditure.

CASE STUDY 4.2
Walking—Solve for the Workload

Jonathan P. is a 34-year-old heart transplant patient whose heart rate varies very little from rest to exercise. He has a $\dot{V}O_2$max of 32 ml·min^{-1}·kg^{-1}. His physician has referred him to your facility for exercise training and wishes him to begin at an intensity between 40% and 60% of $\dot{V}O_2$ reserve. You have found that Mr. P. walks comfortably at 2.5 mph. What treadmill grades would allow him to exercise at the desired intensity range?

First, put all terms into the desired units. Convert the walking speed into m·min^{-1}. Also, determine what values for $\dot{V}O_2$ will be entered into the walking equation using the $\dot{V}O_2$R formula from chapter 2.

$$2.5 \text{ mph} \times 26.8 = 67 \text{ m·min}^{-1}$$
$$\text{Target } \dot{V}O_2 = (\text{intensity fraction})(\dot{V}O_2\text{max} - 3.5) + 3.5$$
$$\text{Lower target } \dot{V}O_2 = (0.40)(32 - 3.5) + 3.5$$
$$= (0.40)(28.5) + 3.5$$
$$= 11.4 + 3.5 \qquad \textit{(continued)}$$

Case Study 4.2   *(continued)*

$$= 14.9 \text{ ml·min}^{-1}\text{·kg}^{-1}$$
$$\text{Upper target } \dot{V}O_2 = (0.60)(32 - 3.5) + 3.5$$
$$= (0.60)(28.5) + 3.5$$
$$= 17.1 + 3.5$$
$$= 20.6 \text{ ml·min}^{-1}\text{·kg}^{-1}$$

Second, select the walking equation from table 4.1, enter the known values, and solve for the unknown grade. Do this twice, once for the lower target and once for the upper target. Doing the lower target first:

$$\dot{V}O_2 = 3.5 + 0.1(\text{speed}) + 1.8(\text{speed})(\text{fractional grade})$$
$$14.9 = 3.5 + 0.1(67) + 1.8(67)(\text{fractional grade})$$

(To solve this equation, first simplify all the terms, doing multiplications first.)

$$14.9 = 3.5 + 6.7 + 120.6(\text{fractional grade})$$

(Continue to simplify, by doing the available addition on the right side of the equation.)

$$14.9 = 10.2 + 120.6(\text{fractional grade})$$

(The terms within the equation cannot be simplified any further. Now isolate the unknown, fractional grade, on its side of the equation. To do this, remove loosely attached terms first—i.e., those that are being added or subtracted with the unknown. Then remove more tightly attached terms—those that are being multiplied or divided with the unknown.)

$$14.9 - 10.2 = 120.6(\text{fractional grade})$$
$$4.7 = 120.6(\text{fractional grade})$$

(Now, remove the 120.6 from the right side of the equation by dividing both sides with that value.)

$$4.7 / 120.6 = \text{fractional grade}$$
$$0.039 = \text{fractional grade}$$
$$\text{or, 3.9\% grade}$$

The lower target $\dot{V}O_2$ would be achieved by walking at 2.5 mph up a treadmill set at approximately 4%. Now, solve for the upper target.

$20.6 = 3.5 + 0.1(67) + 1.8(67)$(fractional grade)

(The right side of the equation was simplified earlier,
so just copy that from above.)

$20.6 = 10.2 + 120.6$(fractional grade)

(Now, solve for the unknown.)

$20.6 - 10.2 = 120.6$(fractional grade)

$10.4 = 120.6$(fractional grade)

$10.4 / 120.6 =$ fractional grade

$0.086 =$ fractional grade

or, 8.6% grade

Mr. P. can achieve the proper intensity in his exercise prescription by walking at 2.5 mph on a treadmill at approximately 4% to 9% grade.

RUNNING

Running on a level surface requires twice the effort as walking, due to the extra work of literally jumping from one foot to the other. To account for this extra work, the horizontal component of the running equation (0.2 ml of O_2 for each m traveled for each kg of body mass) is twice that for walking. In contrast, the vertical component for running up a grade is only half that for walking (0.9 vs. 1.8 ml of O_2 for each kg·m of work).

The difference in the vertical components for walking and running has been a source of confusion. Shouldn't the work of lifting a given amount of body mass a certain distance up a grade be the same, regardless of how one does it? This disparity has often been erroneously explained (and, unfortunately, repeated by the authors [Swain and Leutholtz 1997]!) as an anomaly associated with treadmills: a walker is in constant contact with the treadmill belt, while a runner is airborne between strides, with the treadmill belt sliding beneath. The explanation given was that this loss of contact with the moving belt must mean that the runner wasn't actually climbing as much as a walker on a treadmill or as much as either a walker or a runner on an outdoor hill. Well, this explanation was wrong. A research study, which had been overlooked for several years (Bassett

et al. 1985), compared running up a hill and running up a treadmill—and found that they have the same oxygen cost, which is less
than the vertical component for walking.

So why is the vertical component for running less than it is for
walking? During level running, the runner jumps into the air to land
on the opposite foot. Apparently, some of the vertical movement
that normally occurs during level running is used for the ascent of a
grade. The single equation for running that appears in table 4.1 can
be used for running on a treadmill or for running outdoors. However, it has not been validated for downhill running.

CASE STUDY 4.3

Running—Solve for the $\dot{V}O_2$

Alexandra C. is a 26-year-old, low-risk client who weighs 118 lb.
She is running on a treadmill at 7 mph up a 3% grade. What is her
gross oxygen consumption in METs, and what is her net caloric
expenditure?

First, convert terms into the units used by the metabolic equations.

$$7 \text{ mph} \times 26.8 = 187.6 \text{ m·min}^{-1}$$
$$118 \text{ lb}/2.2 = 53.6 \text{ kg}$$

Second, select the running equation from table 4.1, enter the
known variables, and solve for the unknown $\dot{V}O_2$.

$$\dot{V}O_2 = 3.5 + 0.2(\text{speed}) + 0.9(\text{speed})(\text{fractional grade})$$
$$= 3.5 + 0.2(187.6) + 0.9(187.6)(0.03)$$
$$= 3.5 + 37.52 + 5.0652$$
$$= 46.1 \text{ ml·min}^{-1}·\text{kg}^{-1}$$

Third, convert the answer into the requested terms—i.e., the
gross number of METs and the net kcal·min^{-1}. To convert from
ml·min^{-1}·kg^{-1} to METs, use the conversion factor in table 4.2.

$$(46.1 \text{ ml·min}^{-1}·\text{kg}^{-1})/3.5 = 13.2 \text{ METs}$$

Ms. C. is exercising at 13.2 METs, a little more than 13 times
resting metabolism. To convert from ml·min^{-1}·kg^{-1} to kcal·min^{-1}, use
the intermediate term of L·min^{-1}. But first, subtract 3.5 ml·min^{-1}·kg^{-1},
because the caloric expenditure was requested as a net value.

$$\text{Net } \dot{V}O_2 = 46.1 - 3.5 = 42.6 \text{ ml·min}^{-1}\text{·kg}^{-1}$$

Converting to L·min^{-1}:

$$\frac{(42.6 \text{ ml·min}^{-1}\text{·kg}^{-1})(53.6 \text{ kg})}{1000} = 2.283 \text{ L·min}^{-1}$$

And now, converting to kcal·min^{-1}:

$$2.283 \text{ L·min}^{-1} \times 5 = 11.4 \text{ kcal·min}^{-1}$$

Ms. C. is burning approximately 11.4 kcal·min^{-1} above resting energy expenditure when she runs on a treadmill at 7 mph up a 3% grade.

CASE STUDY 4.4

Running—Solve for the Workload

Jeannie W. is a 57-year-old competitive runner. She is technically in the moderate-risk category because of her age, but she is very fit and healthy, running 50-60 miles per week. Most of her running is on flat ground, and she competes in distance races at a pace of about a 6:30 mile. She would like to know what sort of pace she should try to maintain on a long hill in an upcoming race. The hill has an average grade of 8%. She has a measured $\dot{V}O_2$max of 62 ml·min^{-1}·kg^{-1}. Assuming she can run at 75-85% of $\dot{V}O_2$R for extended periods of time, what speed (and pace per mile) should she anticipate for this hill?

First, you must calculate the value for $\dot{V}O_2$ from the desired percentage of $\dot{V}O_2$R. Do this twice, once for the lower target and once for the upper target.

$$\text{Lower target } \dot{V}O_2 = 0.75(62 - 3.5) + 3.5$$
$$= 0.75(58.5) + 3.5$$
$$= 43.9 + 3.5$$
$$= 47.4 \text{ ml·min}^{-1}\text{·kg}^{-1}$$
$$\text{Upper target } \dot{V}O_2 = 0.85(62 - 3.5) + 3.5$$
$$= 0.85(58.5) + 3.5$$
$$= 49.7 + 3.5$$
$$= 53.2 \text{ ml·min}^{-1}\text{·kg}^{-1} \qquad \textit{(continued)}$$

Case Study 4.4   *(continued)*

Second, select the running equation from table 4.1, enter the known values, and solve for the unknown speed. First, do this for the lower target:

$$\dot{V}O_2 = 3.5 + 0.2(\text{speed}) + 0.9(\text{speed})(\text{fractional grade})$$
$$47.4 = 3.5 + 0.2(\text{speed}) + 0.9(\text{speed})(0.08)$$
$$47.4 = 3.5 + 0.2(\text{speed}) + 0.072(\text{speed})$$
$$47.4 = 3.5 + (0.2 + 0.072)(\text{speed})$$
$$47.4 = 3.5 + 0.272(\text{speed})$$
$$47.4 - 3.5 = 0.272(\text{speed})$$
$$43.9 = 0.272(\text{speed})$$
$$43.9 / 0.272 = \text{speed}$$
$$161.4 \text{ m·min}^{-1} = \text{speed}$$

Now, the upper target:

$$53.2 = 3.5 + 0.2(\text{speed}) + 0.9(\text{speed})(0.08)$$
$$53.2 = 3.5 + 0.272(\text{speed})$$
$$53.2 - 3.5 = 0.272(\text{speed})$$
$$49.7 = 0.272(\text{speed})$$
$$49.7 / 0.272 = \text{speed}$$
$$182.7 \text{ m·min}^{-1} = \text{speed}$$

Third, convert the answer into the desired units—in this case, mph and minutes per mile. To convert from m·min^{-1} to mph, use the conversion factor in table 4.2.

Lower target speed:

$$(161.4 \text{ m·min}^{-1}) / 26.8 = 6.0 \text{ mph}$$

Upper target speed:

$$(182.7 \text{ m·min}^{-1}) / 26.8 = 6.8 \text{ mph}$$

To convert mph to a pace in min per mile, simply divide the mph into 60, and then convert the fractional number of minutes into seconds.

Lower target pace:

$$(60 \text{ min per hr}) / (6.0 \text{ miles per hr}) = 10 \text{ min per mile}$$

Upper target pace:

$$60/6.8 = 8.82 \text{ min per mile}$$
$$= 8 \text{ min} + 0.82 \times 60 \text{ sec per mile}$$
$$= 8 \text{ min and } 49 \text{ sec per mile}$$

Ms. W. can expect to run up the 8% hill at a pace between 8:49 and 10:00, as opposed to her 6:30 pace on flat ground.

LEG CYCLING

As mentioned, the leg cycling equation was modified for the sixth edition of the ACSM's *Guidelines* to include a term for unloaded cycling. Pedaling a bike with no resistance is noticeably more work than sitting still. The mass of the legs is substantial, and moving them in a circle at 50-60 rpm requires about 1 additional MET (i.e., $3.5 \text{ ml}\cdot\text{min}^{-1}\cdot\text{kg}^{-1}$) of oxygen consumption (Lang et al. 1992; Latin and Berg 1994; Londeree et al. 1997). The metabolic equation in table 4.1 has already added the resting and unloaded cycling terms together, yielding a single term of $7 \text{ ml}\cdot\text{min}^{-1}\cdot\text{kg}^{-1}$. The factor for loaded cycling is now 1.8 ml of oxygen for each kg·m of work, which is the same as the value for vertical work in the walking and stepping equations.

Obviously, if people spin their legs faster than 60 rpm, the oxygen cost of unloaded cycling will be higher. However, research has shown that the factor for loaded cycling decreases in a compensating way as cadence increases (Londeree et al. 1997), making the single equation reasonably accurate for cadences up to at least 90 rpm.

Laboratory cycle ergometers generally do not have a power readout but simply indicate the resistance setting (in kg) and the cadence. You can determine the workload, also termed "work rate" for ergometers, from the following equation:

Cycle Ergometry Work Rate Equation

work rate = (resistance setting)(flywheel distance per rev)(rpm)

In this formula, the work rate is in the units $\text{kg}\cdot\text{m}\cdot\text{min}^{-1}$, and the distance that the flywheel travels for one pedal revolution is in meters. This value is 6 m for the Monark leg ergometers and 3 m for

BodyGuard and Tunturi ergometers. Many exercise cycles have a power readout in watts. *One watt is equivalent to approximately 6 kg·m·min⁻¹.*

CASE STUDY 4.5
Leg Cycling—Solve for the $\dot{V}O_2$

Marvin G. is a 37-year-old, 173-lb, moderate-risk client who is exercising to lose weight. He cycles on a Monark ergometer at 50 rpm with a resistance setting of 3 kg. How many minutes would he need to cycle to burn off the calories in one pound of fat?

First, put all of the relevant terms into the units called for by the leg cycling equation. You need to convert the body weight to a body mass and determine the work rate in kg·m·min⁻¹.

$$(173 \text{ lb})/2.2 = 78.6 \text{ kg}$$

Work rate = (resistance setting)(flywheel distance per rev)(rpm)

$$= (3 \text{ kg})(6 \text{ m})(50 \text{ rpm})$$
$$= 900 \text{ kg·m·min}^{-1}$$

Second, select the leg cycling equation from table 4.2, enter the known values, and solve for the unknown $\dot{V}O_2$:

$$\dot{V}O_2 = 7 + 1.8(\text{work rate})/(\text{body mass})$$
$$= 7 + 1.8(900)/78.6$$
$$= 7 + 1620/78.6$$
$$= 7 + 20.6$$
$$= 27.6 \text{ ml·min}^{-1} \cdot \text{kg}^{-1}$$

Third, because the question concerns weight loss, express the $\dot{V}O_2$ as a net value. Then convert it to L·min⁻¹ and finally to kcal·min⁻¹:

$$\text{Net } \dot{V}O_2 = 27.6 - 3.5 = 24.1 \text{ ml·min}^{-1} \cdot \text{kg}^{-1}$$
$$\frac{(24.1 \text{ ml·min}^{-1} \cdot \text{kg}^{-1})(78.6 \text{ kg})}{1000} = 1.894 \text{ L·min}^{-1}$$
$$(1.894 \text{ L·min}^{-1}) \times (5 \text{ kcal·L}^{-1}) = 9.47 \text{ kcal·min}^{-1}$$

One pound of fat contains approximately 3,500 kcal of stored energy, so Mr. G. would need to accumulate 3,500/9.47 = 370 minutes of this exercise (a little over 6 hrs) to lose one pound (assuming all calories burned by the exercise are in excess of dietary intake).

CASE STUDY 4.6
Leg Cycling—Solve for Workload

Abigail R. is a 42-year-old, moderate-risk client who weighs 147 lb. You have estimated her $\dot{V}O_2$max as 29 ml·min^{-1}·kg^{-1} and would like her to exercise at 60-70% of $\dot{V}O_2$R. She has purchased a stationary bike that has a power readout in watts. What would be an appropriate target intensity range for her on this bike?

First, convert terms. In this case, convert her body weight into a body mass, and determine her lower and upper target $\dot{V}O_2$s using the $\dot{V}O_2$R formula:

$$(147 \text{ lb})/2.2 = 66.8 \text{ kg}$$
$$\text{Target } \dot{V}O_2 = (\text{intensity fraction})(\dot{V}O_2\text{max} - 3.5) + 3.5$$
$$\text{Lower target } \dot{V}O_2 = (0.60)(29 - 3.5) + 3.5$$
$$= (0.60)(25.5) + 3.5$$
$$= 15.3 + 3.5$$
$$= 18.8 \text{ ml·min}^{-1}\text{·kg}^{-1}$$
$$\text{Upper target } \dot{V}O_2 = (0.70)(29 - 3.5) + 3.5$$
$$= (0.70)(25.5) + 3.5$$
$$= 17.85 + 3.5$$
$$= 21.4 \text{ ml·min}^{-1}\text{·kg}^{-1}$$

Second, select the leg cycling equation from table 4.1, enter the known values, and solve for the unknown workload:

Lower target workload:

$$\dot{V}O_2 = 7 + 1.8(\text{work rate})/(\text{body mass})$$
$$18.8 = 7 + 1.8(\text{work rate})/66.8$$

(There are three numbers associated with the unknown. To isolate it, remove the most loosely attached term first, the one that is being added.)

$$18.8 - 7 = 1.8(\text{work rate})/66.8$$
$$11.8 = 1.8(\text{work rate})/66.8$$

(continued)

Case Study 4.6 *(continued)*

(Now, remove the other two terms to isolate the unknown. It doesn't matter which is done first. In this example, first multiply both sides by the body mass, and then divide both sides by the work rate coefficient.)

$$11.8 \times 66.8 = 1.8(\text{work rate})$$
$$788.24 = 1.8(\text{work rate})$$
$$788.24 / 1.8 = \text{work rate}$$
$$437.9 \ \text{kg·m·min}^{-1} = \text{work rate}$$

Upper target workload:

$$21.4 = 7 + 1.8(\text{work rate})/66.8$$
$$21.4 - 7 = 1.8(\text{work rate})/66.8$$
$$14.4 = 1.8(\text{work rate})/66.8$$
$$14.4 \times 66.8 = 1.8(\text{work rate})$$
$$961.92 = 1.8(\text{work rate})$$
$$961.92 / 1.8 = \text{work rate}$$
$$534.4 \ \text{kg·m·min}^{-1} = \text{work rate}$$

Third, convert the answer into the desired units. To convert kg·m·min^{-1} to watts, divide the former by 6.

Lower target workload:

$$(437.9 \ \text{kg·m·min}^{-1})/6 = 73 \ \text{W}$$

Upper target workload:

$$(534.4 \ \text{kg·m·min}^{-1})/6 = 89 \ \text{W}$$

Ms. R. can exercise in her target intensity range by cycling at approximately 73-89 watts.

ARM CYCLING

The ACSM's arm cycling metabolic equation does not include a term for unloaded cycling. At this time, available research does not suggest that such a term is needed (Franklin 1985), possibly because of the small mass of the arms as compared to the legs. An important consideration in arm cycling is that it requires significantly more oxygen consumption than leg cycling to perform the same workload, as indicated by the factor of 3 ml of oxygen per kg·m, instead of 1.8 for the legs. It is believed that the higher factor for the arms is due to less efficiency in performing a given amount of work with a smaller muscle mass.

If using a laboratory arm ergometer, always check the flywheel distance before calculating the workload. Monark arm ergometers have a flywheel distance of 2.4 m.

CASE STUDY 4.7
Arm Cycling—Solve for $\dot{V}O_2$

Akiko W. is a 61-year-old, 127-lb, coronary bypass patient. During her phase II rehabilitation, she is introduced to the use of a Monark arm ergometer. She is asked to select a comfortable resistance level while cranking at 50 rpm, keeping her HR within a range prescribed by her physician. After warming up, she uses a resistance of 1 kg. What is her estimated oxygen consumption during this exercise?

First, convert terms to appropriate units. In this case, convert her body weight to body mass, and determine her workload on the arm ergometer in kg·m·min^{-1}:

$$(127 \text{ lb})/2.2 = 57.7 \text{ kg}$$

Work rate = (resistance setting)(flywheel distance per rev)(rpm)

$$= (1 \text{ kg})(2.4 \text{ m})(50 \text{ rpm})$$
$$= 120 \text{ kg·m·min}^{-1}$$

Second, select the arm cycling equation from table 4.1, enter the known values, and solve for the unknown $\dot{V}O_2$:

$$\dot{V}O_2 = 3.5 + 3(\text{work rate})/(\text{body mass})$$
$$= 3.5 + 3(120)/57.7$$
$$= 3.5 + 360/57.7$$
$$= 3.5 + 6.2$$
$$= 9.7 \text{ ml·min}^{-1}\text{·kg}^{-1}$$

Ms. W. is exercising with a gross $\dot{V}O_2$ of approximately 9.7 ml·min^{-1}·kg^{-1} on the arm ergometer.

> ### CASE STUDY 4.8
> ## *Arm Cycling—Solve for the Workload*

Fred J. is an 18-year-old, 152-lb male who had a spinal injury in a car accident six months ago and is now paraplegic. You are prescribing an exercise program for him on a Monark arm ergometer. His $\dot{V}O_2$max (recently measured on an arm ergometer) is 28.5 ml·min^{-1}·kg^{-1}, and you want him to begin his exercise program at 50% of $\dot{V}O_2$R. What is the appropriate workload on the arm ergometer? You have found that he prefers to crank on the ergometer at a cadence of 70 rpm. What resistance setting should be used to achieve the desired workload?

First, convert his body weight into body mass, and determine his target $\dot{V}O_2$ using the $\dot{V}O_2$R formula:

$$(152 \text{ lb})/2.2 = 69.1 \text{ kg}$$

$$\text{Target } \dot{V}O_2 = (\text{intensity fraction})(\dot{V}O_2\text{max} - 3.5) + 3.5$$

$$= (0.50)(28.5 - 3.5) + 3.5$$

$$= (0.50)(25) + 3.5$$

$$= 12.5 + 3.5$$

$$= 16.0 \text{ ml·min}^{-1}\text{·kg}^{-1}$$

Second, select the arm cycling equation from table 4.1, enter the known values, and solve for the unknown workload:

$$\dot{V}O_2 = 3.5 + 3(\text{work rate})/(\text{body mass})$$

$$16.0 = 3.5 + 3(\text{work rate})/69.1$$

$$16.0 - 3.5 = 3(\text{work rate})/69.1$$

$$12.5 = 3(\text{work rate})/69.1$$

$$12.5 \times 69.1 = 3(\text{work rate})$$

$$863.75 = 3(\text{work rate})$$

$$863.75/3 = \text{work rate}$$

$$288 \text{ kg·m·min}^{-1} = \text{work rate}$$

Mr. J.'s workload should be a little less than 290 kg·m·min^{-1}. If he cranks the arm ergometer at 70 rpm, his resistance setting would be as follows:

> Work rate = (resistance setting)(flywheel distance per rev)(rpm)
>
> 288 = (resistance setting)(2.4)(70)
>
> 288 = (resistance setting)(168)
>
> 288 / 168 = resistance setting
>
> 1.7 kg = resistance setting

STEPPING

The ACSM's stepping equation was modified for the 6th edition *Guidelines* to include a term for resting metabolism. The equation is now virtually identical to the original equation established by researchers in 1965 (Nagle, Balke, and Naughton 1965). The oxygen cost for lifting one's body mass up the step is 1.8 ml for each kg·m of work (as in the walking and leg cycling equations). However, one-third must be added to account for the oxygen cost of eccentrically lowering the body mass back down. Thus, the equation in table 4.1 uses a factor of 2.4, i.e., 1.8 + (1/3 of 1.8).

The stepping rate in the equation refers to complete four-cycle steps per minute: (1) lift the first leg onto the bench; (2) step up and place the second leg on the bench; (3) step down with the first leg; (4) step down with the second leg. There are four movements making up one "step," so set your metronome at four times the desired stepping rate to help your clients stay on cadence. The first leg is doing all of the concentric (lifting) work and the second leg is doing all the eccentric (lowering) work, so instruct clients to switch legs occasionally. They can do this by tapping the second leg on the floor at the end of a cycle and immediately lifting it back onto the step.

CASE STUDY 4.9
Stepping—Solve for the $\dot{V}O_2$

Kathy M. is a 46-year-old aerobic dance instructor. During her stepping classes, she leads her clients in a routine performed at 20 steps per minute (to a beat of 80 min^{-1}). If the class is using 4-inch benches, what is their estimated $\dot{V}O_2$ in ml·min^{-1}·kg^{-1} and in METs?

(continued)

Case Study 4.9   *(continued)*

First, convert terms. The step height must be entered into the equation in meters. One inch is equal to 2.54 cm, or to 0.0254 m.

$$(4 \text{ inches}) \times 0.0254 = 0.10 \text{ m}$$

Second, select the stepping equation from table 4.1, enter the known values, and solve for the unknown $\dot{V}O_2$:

$$\dot{V}O_2 = 3.5 + 0.2(\text{stepping rate}) + 2.4(\text{stepping rate})(\text{step height})$$
$$= 3.5 + 0.2(20) + 2.4(20)(0.10)$$
$$= 3.5 + 4.0 + 4.8$$
$$= 12.3 \text{ ml·min}^{-1}\text{·kg}^{-1}$$

Third, convert to the desired units.

$$(12.3 \text{ ml·min}^{-1}\text{·kg}^{-1})/3.5 = 3.5 \text{ METs}$$

CASE STUDY 4.10
Stepping—Solve for the Workload

One member of Ms. M.'s stepping class, Sheri C., has purchased a set of stackable benches for use at home. The benches come in 2-inch increments and can be stacked to a height of 10 inches. Sheri C. is 32 years old, weighs 128 lb, and is in the low-risk category. Her $\dot{V}O_2$max has been estimated as 38 ml·min^{-1}·kg^{-1}. To exercise at 70% of $\dot{V}O_2$R, what stepping rate would she need on the 10-inch bench? At what rate should she set her metronome?

First, convert the bench height to meters, and determine the target $\dot{V}O_2$ from the $\dot{V}O_2$R formula:

$$(10 \text{ inches}) \times 0.0254 = 0.254 \text{ m}$$
$$\text{Target } \dot{V}O_2 = (\text{intensity fraction})(\dot{V}O_2\text{max} - 3.5) + 3.5$$
$$= (0.70)(38 - 3.5) + 3.5$$
$$= (0.70)(34.5) + 3.5$$
$$= 24.15 + 3.5$$
$$= 27.7 \text{ ml·min}^{-1}\text{·kg}^{-1}$$

Second, select the stepping equation from table 4.1, enter the known values, and solve for the unknown stepping rate:

$$\dot{V}O_2 = 3.5 + 0.2(\text{stepping rate}) + 2.4(\text{stepping rate})(\text{step height})$$
$$27.7 = 3.5 + 0.2(\text{stepping rate}) + 2.4(\text{stepping rate})(0.254)$$
$$27.7 = 3.5 + 0.2(\text{stepping rate}) + 0.6096(\text{stepping rate})$$
$$27.7 = 3.5 + (0.2 + 0.6096)(\text{stepping rate})$$
$$27.7 = 3.5 + 0.8096(\text{stepping rate})$$
$$27.7 - 3.5 = 0.8096(\text{stepping rate})$$
$$24.2 = 0.8096(\text{stepping rate})$$
$$24.2 / 0.8096 = \text{stepping rate}$$
$$29.89 \text{ steps} \cdot \text{min}^{-1} = \text{stepping rate}$$

The stepping rate for Ms. C. should be 30 steps per minute. She should set her metronome at four times this, or 120 bpm.

REFERENCES

1. Bassett, DR, MD Giese, FJ Nagle, A Ward, DM Raab, and B Balke. 1985. Aerobic requirements of overground versus treadmill running. *Med. Sci. Sports Exerc.* 17:477-481.

2. Franklin, BA. 1985. Exercise testing, training and arm ergometry. *Sports Med.* 2:100-119.

3. Franklin, BA, ed. 2000. *ACSM's Guidelines for Exercise Testing and Prescription*, 6th ed., 300-312. Philadelphia: Lippincott Williams & Wilkins.

4. Lang, PB, RW Latin, KE Berg, and MB Mellion. 1992. The accuracy of the ACSM cycle ergometry equation. *Med. Sci. Sports Exerc.* 24:272-276.

5. Latin, RW, and KE Berg. 1994. The accuracy of the ACSM and a new cycle ergometry equation for young women. *Med. Sci. Sports Exerc.* 26:642-646.

6. Londeree, BR, J Moffitt-Gerstenberger, JA Padfield, and D Lottmann. 1997. Oxygen consumption of cycle ergometry is nonlinearly related to work rate and pedal rate. *Med. Sci. Sport Exerc.* 29:775-780.

7. Nagle, FJ, B Balke, and JP Naughton. 1965. Gradational step tests for assessing work capacity. *J. Appl. Physiol.* 20:745-748.

8. Swain, DP. 2000. Energy cost calculations for exercise prescription: an update. *Sports Med.* 30:17-22.

9. Swain, DP, and BC Leutholtz. 1997. *Metabolic Calculations—Simplified*, 73. Baltimore: Williams & Wilkins.

CHAPTER

5

Exercise Prescription for Weight Loss

Approximately 300,000 adult Americans die each year from obesity-related diseases. Obesity is a major risk factor for chronic disease, and it results in substantial health care costs. Currently, obesity continues to increase in Americans across all sociodemographic groups and in all parts of the United States. It has been conservatively estimated that there are between 5 and 10 million obese Americans (Allison et al. 1999). Prevalence rates for obesity have increased by 57% since 1991, along with an approximate 33% increase in diabetes (Mokdad et al. 1999). Americans between the ages of 18 and 29 reported the largest increases in body weight. Most experts recognize that the prevalence of obesity is likely to increase in the future.

Obesity may or may not be a health risk in and of itself. However, when body fat percentages exceed 25 and 30 percent in sedentary males and females, respectively, or body mass index exceeds 30 kg·m^{-2}, the risk for hypokinetic diseases—such as heart disease, high blood pressure, and diabetes—may increase. Currently, about 25-30% of Americans are considered at risk as a result of excessive body fat (Franklin 2000). Furthermore, even with all the low-fat and nonfat food choices, this percentage is increasing as advancing technology creates a more sedentary society.

ENERGY BALANCE

People gain weight when they achieve a positive caloric balance—i.e., when they consume more calories than they expend. Figure 5.1 illustrates various sources of energy intake and energy expenditure. Energy intake is approximately 4 kcal per gram of carbohydrates or protein, 7 kcal per gram of ethyl alcohol, and 9 kcal per gram of fat. The actual energy values for these chemical substances are somewhat higher, but the amount absorbed by the body is less than the amount actually eaten; and, in the case of proteins, a portion of the caloric value is lost when amino acids are deaminated for caloric use.

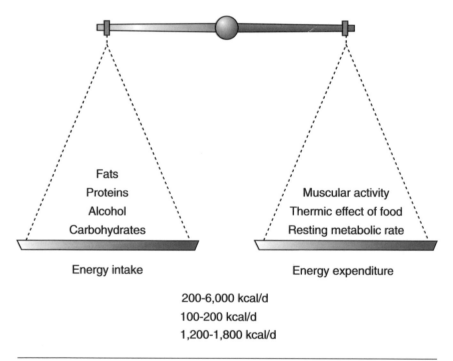

Fats
Proteins
Alcohol
Carbohydrates

Muscular activity
Thermic effect of food
Resting metabolic rate

Energy intake   Energy expenditure

200-6,000 kcal/d
100-200 kcal/d
1,200-1,800 kcal/d

Figure 5.1   Energy balance is determined by caloric intake from various food sources vs. energy expenditure. Resting metabolic rate and the thermic effect of food are relatively fixed values, but energy expenditure from muscular activity varies tremendously based on an individual's personal choices. If energy expenditure exceeds intake, weight loss will occur.

Energy expenditure is due to resting metabolic rate (RMR), the thermic effect of food, and muscular activity. **Resting metabolic rate** is approximately 1 kcal per hour for each kilogram of body mass. However, it is lower for individuals with a high proportion of body fat, since adipose tissue has a lower metabolic rate than does lean tissue. The digestion and assimilation of food is an energy-requiring process known as the **thermic effect of food,** and it expends 5-10% of the calories consumed. The most variable source of energy expenditure is muscular activity. Sedentary individuals may expend no more than 200 to 300 kcal per day in activities of daily living, and individuals with physically demanding jobs or who engage in structured exercise might expend several hundred, and up to a few thousand, additional kcal per day. Competitors in the Tour de France bicycle race need to consume 6,000-8,000 kcal per day to maintain caloric balance.

If an individual is in a positive energy balance, the excess calories will be stored in the body. Carbohydrates can be stored as glycogen, but total body stores of glycogen are only 1,000-2,000 kcal. Once glycogen stores are filled, any excessive carbohydrate consumption will be converted to fat and stored as adipose tissue. Proteins can be "stored" as muscle tissue but only if the individual is engaged in a properly structured resistance training program. Even then, the rate of muscular growth is very slow, especially in highly trained subjects, being only a few pounds per year under the best conditions. Therefore, most protein intake that exceeds daily needs is converted to fat and stored as adipose tissue. Any alcohol or fat that is consumed in excess of immediate caloric needs is also stored as adipose tissue. The body is well designed to store any source of excess calories as fat, as a protection against famine. In modern society, this storage of fat is generally unnecessary and is clearly not worth the risk of associated chronic diseases.

WEIGHT MANAGEMENT

Body composition can be measured by a variety of methods, some better than others. For example, methods that distinguish between body fat and lean muscle are regarded as the best because a person can be overweight without being overfat. A very athletic or muscular individual might fall into the "overweight" category.

A specific cause for obesity is yet to be discovered. It appears to be multifactorial in nature, with inactivity being a leading component.

Therefore, therapy should address behavioral, social, and cultural factors. Long-term medications for the treatment of obesity are not available. Current medications include sympathomimetics and serotonin inhibitors. These medications appear to result in weight loss—yet for safety concerns, their long-term use is not recommended and weight gain usually returns when the medications are discontinued. Unfortunately, the failure or recidivism rate for weight loss programs is approximately 70-95% (Leutholtz and Ripoll 1999).

The ACSM recommends a balanced approach to weight loss that results in gradual body fat loss of no more than 1 kg per week (Franklin 2000). This should be accomplished by achieving a negative caloric balance of 500-1000 kcal per day, with at least 300 kcal of this negative balance coming from daily exercise. Rapid weight loss accomplished by drastically reducing caloric intake should be avoided.

In your exercise prescriptions, emphasize duration and frequency (progressing to one hour daily) over intensity, until your client can exercise at an intensity suitable for cardiovascular conditioning. You should also instruct your client in proper eating habits—i.e., consuming a well-balanced diet that is low in fat and moderately reduced in total calories.

EXERCISE PRESCRIPTION FOR FAT LOSS

In designing exercise prescriptions for reducing body fat, always consider the four basic variables of aerobic exercise—frequency, intensity, time (duration), and type. Once your client has settled into a regular program of aerobic exercise, you can add weightlifting to the program. However, the initial focus should be on increasing the volume of exercise and caloric expenditure, which can best be achieved by doing aerobic exercise. Resistance training can result in a small increase in lean body mass, which will increase caloric expenditure by increasing resting metabolism, but this effect is comparatively small.

An important consideration in prescribing exercise is to recognize that only the *net* caloric expenditure can be counted toward fat loss. The net caloric expenditure is that which is due to the exercise itself, whereas the gross caloric expenditure is the net value plus the amount associated with rest. The resting caloric expenditure should not be counted toward fat loss (unless the client is fasting), since the client would burn those same calories whether or not he or she was exercising.

Exercise is critical for properly achieving a negative caloric balance. However, sedentary individuals are not capable of performing at a high rate of energy expenditure, and thus must accumulate a large total duration on a weekly basis to effectively lose fat weight. For example, walking at 3.5 mph (about a 17 minute per mile pace) burns only 3.3 kcal per minute above resting energy expenditure for a 70-kg client (a heavier client would burn proportionally more). If the same individual could run at 7 mph (about an 8½ minute per mile pace), he or she would burn calories four times faster. For each mile covered, the runner burns twice as many calories as the walker and is covering miles twice as fast, thus accounting for the fourfold greater rate of expenditure. Note: A common error is to assume that walking and running burn the same number of calories per mile, often estimated as 100 kcal. However, this refers to the *gross* number

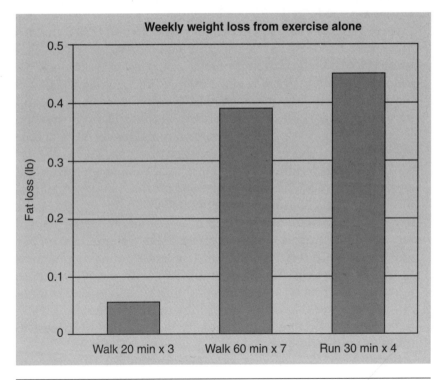

Figure 5.2 The amount of fat that would be lost by exercise alone (assuming no increase in caloric consumption) by a 70-kg (154-lb) person. Fat loss by heavier individuals would be proportionally greater. "Walking" is at 3.5 mph, burning a net 3.3 kcal per minute. "Running" is at 7.0 mph, burning a net 13.1 kcal per minute.

of calories, including those due to resting metabolism. Since walkers take longer to cover the mile, they burn more calories associated with the resting component than runners do, resulting in similar totals per mile. For weight loss purposes, however, only the net caloric expenditure should be counted. As figure 5.2 illustrates, walkers would need a little over an hour of exercise 7 days per week to lose ½ lb of fat, whereas runners would obtain as much weight loss with only 30 minutes of exercise, 4 days a week.

CASE STUDY 5.1
Weight Loss Client

Arthur W. is a sedentary 40-year-old man who has been gradually gaining weight for the last ten years. Mr. W. recently saw his medical doctor for a routine physical. His current weight and height are 250 lb and 5'9". His body mass index is 37 $kg \cdot m^{-2}$. He reported that he was experiencing chest pain and stated that his brother had a heart attack when he was 47. His physician performed a maximal cardiopulmonary stress test and obtained the following results: $\dot{V}O_2max$ of 30 $ml \cdot min^{-1} \cdot kg^{-1}$, maximal HR 170 bpm, resting HR 90 bpm, normal ECG response to exercise, and no signs or symptoms of heart disease. His physician advised him to begin a weight loss program with an initial loss of 50 lb, and he referred him to you to begin an exercise program.

Mr. W.'s goal weight is 200 lb. He is very anxious to lose weight and wants to reach his goal in just one month. However, you remind him that it has taken him 10 years to gain this weight, and a loss of 2 lb per week would result in a safer and more permanent reduction in about six months. You decide that stepping exercises and jogging are too rigorous for a sedentary overweight individual. After discussing the other options with Mr. W., you both agree that the best type of exercise for him is walking and stationary cycling. You ask Mr. W. to begin with 20-30 minutes of walking every other day and to gradually increase this to at least 45 minutes on a daily basis.

Because Mr. W. has been sedentary for the last 10 years, you choose a fairly low to moderate window for his intensity—perhaps 50-70% of heart rate reserve, or $\dot{V}O_2R$. Since Mr. W. had a maximal stress test, in your calculations you can use his measured maximum HR of 170 beats per minute. Calculate a target heart rate at 50% and 70% of Mr. W.'s heart rate reserve.

Target HR = (intensity fraction)(HRmax − HRrest) + HRrest

Lower target HR = (0.5)(170 − 90) + 90

= (0.5)(80) + 90

= 40 + 90

= 130 bpm

Upper target HR = (0.7)(170 − 90) + 90

= (0.7)(80) + 90

= 56 + 90

= 146 bpm

Next, Mr. W. tells you that he has to walk a brisk 3.7 mph on a treadmill at 0% grade to reach the lower end of his heart rate prescription of 130 bpm. How many calories is he burning at this point? To determine this, first calculate his $\dot{V}O_2$ using the walking equation from table 4.1. Table 4.2 indicates that, to convert mph to m·min^{-1} multiply by 26.8. Thus, the speed is (3.7 mph) × 26.8 = 99.2 m·min^{-1}.

$\dot{V}O_2$ = 3.5 + 0.1(speed) + 1.8(speed)(fractional grade)

= 3.5 + 0.1(99.2) + 1.8(99.2)(0)

= 3.5 + 9.92 + 0

= 13.4 ml·min^{-1}·kg^{-1} (gross $\dot{V}O_2$)

net $\dot{V}O_2$ = 13.4 − 3.5 = 9.9 ml·min^{-1}·kg^{-1}

(Note that this is less than 50% of his $\dot{V}O_2$R. This workload was chosen on the basis of his target HR, and target HRs and target $\dot{V}O_2$s will not always match, because both are estimates of his actual physiological responses.)

Now, convert to caloric expenditure by using the conversion formulas in table 4.2. First, convert $\dot{V}O_2$ in ml·min^{-1}·kg^{-1} to L·min^{-1}; then convert the $\dot{V}O_2$ to kcal·min^{-1}.

(9.9 ml·min^{-1}·kg^{-1})(113.6 kg)/1000 = 1.12 L·min^{-1}

Next, remember that 5 kilocalories are expended for each liter of oxygen consumed; therefore, during a 45-minute exercise session, Mr. W. would burn the following number of calories:

(1.12 L·min^{-1}) × (5 kcal·L^{-1}) = 5.6 kcal·min^{-1}

(5.6 kcal·min^{-1}) × (45 minutes) = 252 kcal per session

(continued)

Case Study 5.1   *(continued)*

Finally, do one more calculation with Mr. W. Three months have passed, and as a result of Mr. W.'s exercise and dietary changes he has lost 25 pounds, and is now able to jog and achieve the upper end of his target heart rate range, 146 bpm. To achieve this heart rate he tells you that he must now jog at 4.5 mph. He has not been able to increase his exercise session from 45 minutes but wants to know how many calories he is burning. To calculate this figure, use the running equation from table 4.1. His speed is (4.5 mph) $\times$ 26.8 = 120.6 m·min^{-1}.

$$\dot{V}O_2 = 3.5 + 0.2(\text{speed}) + 0.9(\text{speed})(\text{fractional grade})$$
$$\dot{V}O_2 = 3.5 + 0.2(120.6) + 0.9(120.6)(0)$$
$$= 3.5 + 24.12 + 0$$
$$\dot{V}O_2 = 27.6 \text{ ml·min}^{-1}\text{·kg}^{-1} \text{ (gross } \dot{V}O_2)$$
$$\text{net } \dot{V}O_2 = 27.6 - 3.5 = 24.1 \text{ ml·min}^{-1}\text{·kg}^{-1}$$

(Note that this is more than 70% of $\dot{V}O_2R$ based on his original $\dot{V}O_2$max. However, his aerobic capacity has improved and, as noted earlier, his workloads based on HR and based on $\dot{V}O_2$ will not match precisely.)

Convert to L·min^{-1} and then to kcal·min^{-1}. Note that his new body mass is (225 lb)/2.2 = 102.3 kg:

$$(24.1 \text{ ml·min}^{-1}\text{·kg}^{-1}) \times (102.3 \text{ kg})/1000 = 2.47 \text{ L·min}^{-1}$$
$$(2.47 \text{ L·min}^{-1}) \times (5 \text{ kcal·L}^{-1}) = 12.3 \text{ kcal·min}^{-1}$$
$$(12.3 \text{ kcal·min}^{-1}) \times (45 \text{ minutes}) = 554 \text{ kcal per session}$$

Mr. W. has doubled his caloric expenditure by increasing his intensity or speed.

Mr. W.'s exercise prescription can be summarized as follows:

Frequency: A minimum of five days per week to maximize caloric expenditure.

Intensity: A target heart rate range of 130-146 beats per minute, to place him at approximately 50-70% of $\dot{V}O_2R$. If an individual is not able to maintain a target heart rate continuously, the intensity should be decreased and the time increased to maintain caloric expenditure.

Time: Mr. W. requires at least 45 minutes of exercise to achieve the recommended 300-500 kilocalorie expenditure per exercise session.

Type: You have prescribed modalities that exercise large muscle groups, such as walking and cycling, in order to maximize caloric expenditure. (Note that nonweightbearing activities are recommended for people with orthopedic concerns.)

CASE STUDY 5.2
Weight Loss Client

Look at another client, Sheila K., who is obese with a body fat percentage of 37%, measured by the underwater weighing or hydrodensitometry method. Her current weight is 205 pounds, she is 5'5" tall, and her age is 32. Her body mass index (BMI) is 34 kg·m^{-2}. Ms. K. has osteoarthritis but does not have a significant history of, or risk factors for, heart disease. Ms. K. has been referred to you by her physician for an exercise program designed to help her lose weight.

Because Ms. K. has two ACSM risk factors—obesity and sedentary behavior—she is in the moderate-risk category. Yet she already has her physician's recommendation that she exercise. As a starting point, Ms. K. agrees to a goal of reaching 30% fat. To determine her goal weight at this level, use the following formula. In the formula, %fat must be entered as a fraction.

$$\text{goal weight} = \frac{(\text{current weight})(1 - \text{current \%fat})}{(1 - \text{desired \%fat})}$$

$$\text{goal weight} = (205)(1 - 0.37)/(1 - 0.30)$$

$$= (205)(0.63)/(0.70)$$

= 129/0.70 (i.e., her lean body weight is 129 lb, and we would like this to be 70% of her total, instead of 63%)

$$= 184 \text{ lb}$$

Now that an initial goal weight for Ms. K. has been determined, develop her exercise prescription. Because of her arthritis, she might use a stationary bike for the mode of exercise. She agrees to

(continued)

Case Study 5.2 *(continued)*

exercise at least five days per week and to gradually increase her duration to one hour per session. You have decided to set the intensity level at 50% and 75% of $\dot{V}O_2R$, using the heart rate reserve method. Having instructed Ms. K. to take her resting heart rate when she wakes up in the morning, you estimate her maximal heart rate using the calculation 220 – age. Her resting heart rate is reported to be 85 bpm, and her estimated maximal heart rate is 220 – 32 = 188 bpm. Now calculate her target heart rate range:

$$\text{Target HR} = (\text{intensity fraction})(\text{HRmax} - \text{HRrest}) + \text{HRrest}$$
$$\text{Lower target HR} = (0.5)(188 - 85) + 85$$
$$= (0.5)(103) + 85$$
$$= 51.5 + 85$$
$$= 136 \text{ bpm}$$
$$\text{Upper target HR} = (0.7)(188 - 85) + 85$$
$$= (0.7)(103) + 85$$
$$= 72 + 85$$
$$= 157 \text{ bpm}$$

Ms. K. tells you that to exercise in her heart rate range of 136-157, she must pedal her stationary bike at 75 watts or 450 kg·m·min^{-1} (one watt is approximately equal to 6 kg·m·min^{-1}). First calculate her $\dot{V}O_2$ at this intensity using the cycling equation from table 4.1.

$$\dot{V}O_2 = 7 + 1.8(\text{work rate})/(\text{body mass})$$
$$= 7 + 1.8(450)/93.2$$
$$= 7 + 810/93.2$$
$$= 7 + 8.7$$
$$= 15.7 \text{ ml·min}^{-1}\text{·kg}^{-1} \text{ (gross } \dot{V}O_2)$$
$$\text{net } \dot{V}O_2 = 15.7 - 3.5 = 12.2 \text{ ml·min}^{-1}\text{·kg}^{-1}$$

Convert your answer to liters per minute and multiply by 5 to calculate how many kilocalories Ms. K. is expending per minute of exercise. (Remember to use *net* $\dot{V}O_2$.)

$$(12.2 \text{ ml·min}^{-1}\text{·kg}^{-1}) \times (93.2 \text{ kg})/1000 = 1.14 \text{ L·min}^{-1}$$
$$(1.14 \text{ L·min}^{-1}) \times (5 \text{ kcal·L}^{-1}) = 5.7 \text{ kcal·min}^{-1}$$
$$(5.7 \text{ kcal·min}^{-1})(60 \text{ min}) = 342 \text{ kcal per session}$$

Ms. K. has a current weight of 205 lb and a goal weight of 184 lb, for a total weight loss of 21 lb. Remind her that an appropriate amount of weight to lose is no more than 1 kg per week, or approximately 2 lb. At that rate, it will take Ms. K. about 10 weeks to reach her goal weight. If she exercised five days per week for 60 minutes, she would expend $342 \times 5 = 1710$ *net* kilocalories per week as a result of exercise. However, remember that 2 lb of fat contains 7,000 kilocalories. Therefore, to lose 2 lb per week, the remaining 5290 kilocalorie reduction each week (or $5290/7 = 756$ kcal per day) should come from a modification in her diet. You might consider recommending a consultation with a registered dietitian for Ms. K.

REFERENCES

1. Allison, DB, KR Fontaine, JE Manson, J Stevens, and TB VanItallie. 1999. Annual deaths attributable to obesity in the United States. *J. Am. Med. Assoc.* 282:1530-1538.

2. Franklin, BA, ed. 2000. *ACSM's Guidelines for Exercise Testing and Prescription*, 6th ed., 214-216. Philadelphia: Lippincott Williams & Wilkins.

3. Leutholtz, BC, and I Ripoll. 1999. *Exercise and Disease Management*, ed. I Wolinsky, 97-104. Boca Raton: CRC Press.

4. Mokdad, AH, MK Serdula, WH Dietz, BA Bowman, JS Marks, and JP Koplan. 1999. The spread of the obesity epidemic in the United States, 1991-1998. *J. Am. Med. Assoc.* 282:1519-1522.

6

Exercise Prescription for Muscular Strength and Flexibility

What defines a "fit" person? If this question had been asked back in the early 1900s, the answer might have been "someone who can chop a cord of wood." The answer in the 1940s might have been "an individual with huge muscles, like Charles Atlas." In the 1970s one might answer, "someone who, like my neighbor, runs every morning and competes in weekend marathons." The definition of fitness has evolved over the past century. Today, being fit only aerobically or only in terms in muscle strength does not account for overall fitness. People should strive for optimum function in all components of fitness to achieve total body health. This chapter focuses on resistance training and flexibility guidelines as part of total fitness.

FLEXIBILITY

Flexibility involves moving a joint through its entire range of motion. Having good flexibility is important not only in athletic performance, but also for everyday activities. All exercise programs should include flexibility exercises that promote the improvement or maintenance of flexibility. Lack of flexibility is associated with back pain and a reduced ability to perform activities of daily living.

When to Stretch

Stretching is a very important part of an exercise prescription that is often neglected or performed improperly. Ideally, stretching should be done when the core temperature of the muscle is sufficiently warmed up. For warming to occur, the muscle must be actively contracted. Although sitting in the sun or a hot tub may make you feel warm because the core temperature of your body rises, this does not properly warm up the skeletal muscles in preparation for exercise. The safest time to stretch is during the warm-down following an aerobic or resistance exercise session, when the muscles are still warm. However, stretching also may be included at the end of the warm-up for an exercise session, or done at a separate time as long as a specific warm-up is performed for the stretching session itself.

Flexibility in the lower back and posterior thigh regions is particularly important to decrease the risk for lower back injuries and pain. A regular stretching program may reduce the decline in flexibility that occurs with aging, and it may improve balance, especially for older adults. Flexibility is joint-specific, so no single stretch can achieve total body flexibility.

Types of Stretches

There are three different types or categories of stretches—static, ballistic, and proprioceptive neuromuscular facilitation (PNF). Static stretches are the preferred method for most individuals to maintain or improve range of motion in a joint. The risk of injury is lowest, and it requires little time and assistance to be effective.

How to Stretch

In **static stretching,** the muscle group is slowly stretched to the point of tension or mild discomfort and held for 10-30 seconds. Each stretch should be performed for three or four repetitions to obtain the best results. The frequency of stretching should be at least two to three days per week and can be performed on a daily basis. See figures 6.1-6.5 for examples of static stretches.

The second type of stretch is the ballistic stretch. The **ballistic stretch** is a "dynamic" stretch because it involves active bouncing movements. When this stretch is performed too aggressively, it can injure the connective tissue if the joint's range of motion is exceeded. Furthermore, if the muscle is suddenly stretched very forcefully, a reflex contraction may occur that can actually shorten the muscle and inhibit the stretch. The ballistic stretch may have a place in the warm-up, *provided the type of movements performed during the workout are similar to the stretch;* however, the ACSM does not recommend use of the ballistic stretch.

The final type of stretch is **proprioceptive neuromuscular facilitation,** or the **PNF stretch.** The PNF stretch has been reported to

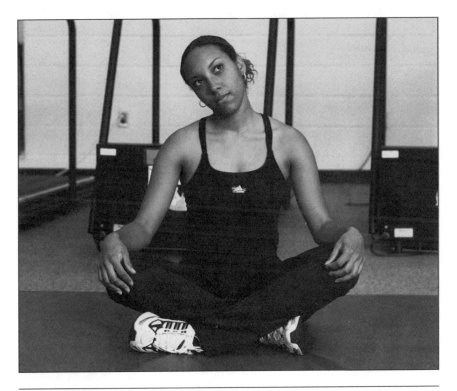

Figure 6.1   Neck stretch (muscles of the neck). Gently move your head from side to side so that the ear moves toward the shoulder. Then move your head forward and back so that the chin drops down toward the chest and then the head returns to a vertical position. Do not hyperextend the neck back or do complete circles in a rapid motion.

produce the greatest improvements in flexibility (Pollock et al. 1998). However, it can cause muscle soreness. Doing this type of stretch involves contracting and relaxing opposing muscle groups with the assistance of a partner. This stretch can be demonstrated by having a client lie on his back on a table and lifting one leg up into the air. A partner places his shoulder under the client's calf to prepare to push the leg farther up. Before this is done, the client pushes down against the partner's shoulder with his leg to forcefully contract his ham-

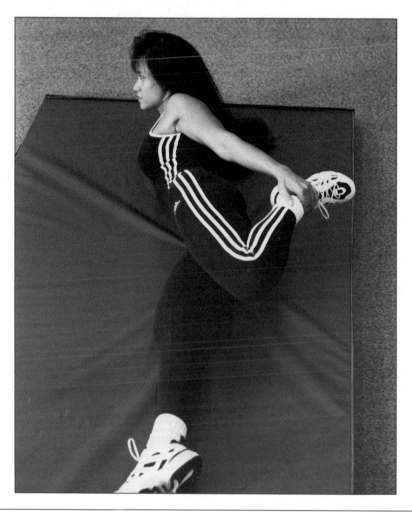

Figure 6.2   Quadriceps stretch (muscles of the anterior thigh). Gently pull your ankle toward your gluteals. When you feel tension, hold. Avoid pulling the heel tight against the gluteals; rather pull the entire leg back.

strings and gluteals. This contraction is held for six seconds. At the moment the client ceases the contraction, the partner pushes the leg farther up, resulting in a greater stretch of the muscles. This stretch can be further enhanced through the process of **reciprocal inhibition** in which the client forcefully contracts the antagonist muscles, in this case the quadriceps, during the stretch. As with static stretching, PNF stretches should be held for 10-30 seconds, performed for three to four repetitions, and be done at least two to three times per week.

Figures 6.1-6.5 provide some examples of static stretches. If you are interested in a more comprehensive listing of stretching exercises, see the National Strength and Conditioning Association's 2nd edition of *Essentials of Strength Training and Conditioning* (Baechle and Earle 2000).

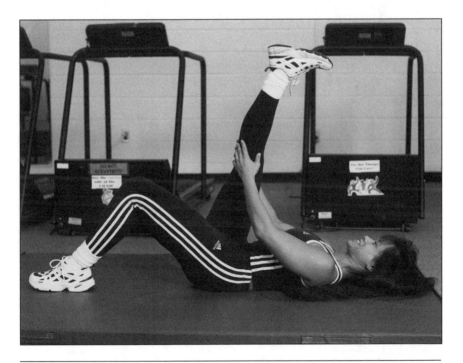

Figure 6.3 Hamstring stretch (muscles of the posterior thigh). Lie flat on your back with your knees bent. Extend one leg with your hands cupped behind your knee, and gently pull. Keep the hands behind the knee to avoid stress on the knee. If performing this stretch in a seated position, do not curve the trunk downward (instead, keep the back relatively straight) and do not bend the opposite knee in the "hurdler's" position.

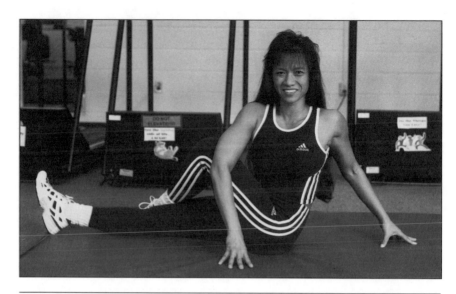

Figure 6.4 Sit-and-twist (muscles of the trunk and back). Sitting on the floor, bend the left leg and cross it over the right leg. Place your right elbow across your body outside your left thigh and your left hand on the floor behind you; slowly rotate to the left and then hold. Repeat in mirror image for the opposite side.

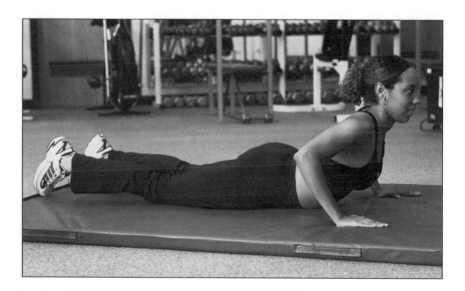

Figure 6.5 Back hypertension stretch (muscles of the lower back and abdomen). Lie prone on the floor. With arms extended and palms flat on the floor, slowly arch your chest and hold. Do not push the waist up off the floor.

MUSCULAR STRENGTH

Muscular strength refers to the greatest force that can be generated by a specific muscle group or groups. It can be measured by a variety of devices such as handgrip dynamometers and cable tensiometers, or by performing or estimating a one-repetition maximum (1-RM). **Muscular endurance** is the ability to perform multiple repetitions at a given percentage of 1-RM. Individuals with a high degree of muscular strength can perform activities of daily living, as well as athletic pursuits, at lower percentages of 1-RM, and thus with less relative effort.

Resistance Training Guidelines

The major benefits of resistance training include maintaining or increasing muscular strength and endurance, muscle mass, bone density, and metabolic rate. Skeletal muscles adapt or improve their size and strength when an overload is applied. This overload can be accomplished by increasing the **intensity** (i.e., the resistance or weight), **duration** (number of sets performed), or **frequency** of the workouts. One complete repetition of a lift involves two phases. First is the **concentric** phase, when the muscle shortens as it applies force to lift the weight. Second is the **eccentric** phase when the weight is returned to its starting position. During the eccentric phase, the muscle is still applying force, but it is being lengthened. Dynamic resistance programs that include both concentric and eccentric components are of the greatest benefit. Routines that emphasize the eccentric component may increase muscle soreness.

The number of repetitions to fatigue determines the *intensity* of resistance exercise. Lifting a weight that fatigues the muscle after 8-12 repetitions develops muscular strength *and* endurance. For most exercises, this occurs with a weight that is approximately 80% of the maximal lift (i.e., 80% of the one-repetition maximum, or 1-RM). The greatest increases in strength occur when a person lifts heavier weights that produce fatigue with fewer than 8 repetitions; to build muscular endurance, however, one should use lower weights and at least 12 repetitions per set (Pollock et al. 1998). Thus, the 8-12 RM range is a compromise intended to improve both strength and muscular endurance.

You can determine the weight that represents 8-12 RM for a client in two ways. One way is simply trial and error. Begin with a very light weight and ask the client to perform 12 repetitions. If she can do this without complete fatigue on the last repetition, increase the weight until she can perform at least 8 repetitions but no more than 12. Alternatively, you can determine the 1-RM (also by trial and error) and then use 80% of this value in the first training session. If this weight causes fatigue in less than 8 repetitions, reduce it; if your client can perform more than 12 repetitions with this weight, increase it. Continue to adjust the weight until fatigue occurs within the 8-12 repetition range. Performing a 1-RM test on older individuals (greater than 50-60 years of age) is not recommended. Once the 8-12 RM is established by either technique, clients enter the progressive phase of training in which the weight is increased by about 10% whenever they reach 12 repetitions.

The *time*, or duration, of a resistance training workout depends on the number of exercises performed and the number of sets performed for each exercise. The ACSM recommends that beginning lifters perform 8-10 different exercises that train all of the major muscle groups in a single exercise session. At least one set of each exercise should be performed. Multiple sets may produce somewhat greater gains, but the total duration of the workout session should be no more than one hour. Longer sessions may result in client attrition.

The ACSM recommends a *frequency* of two or three resistance training sessions per week. These sessions should occur on alternate days, allowing at least 48 hours of recovery time between workouts. Individuals performing more advanced routines may utilize multiple sets and exercises for specific muscle groups—in which case they typically split the routine into two or more parts, and perform each part only two days per week.

Resistance Training Technique

It is critical that you teach clients proper weightlifting technique to optimize strength gains and to ensure their safety.

The components of proper weightlifting form are full range of motion (ROM), isolation, controlled movement speed, and proper breathing.

▶ **Full Range of Motion.** Each lift should be performed through the greatest ROM available for the joint or joints being targeted by the exercise. Partial movements will result in adaptations specific to the limited range that was used.

▶ **Isolation.** Each lift should be performed so that only the target muscles contribute to the movement. Use of accessory muscles (so called "cheating" movements) is common among lifters who are motivated solely to increase the weight. A greater training effect of the target muscles will occur when they are maximally stimulated and not assisted by other muscle groups. Examples of cheating are arching the back during a bench press and swaying the torso backward during a biceps curl.

▸ **Controlled Movement Speed.** The speed of movement throughout an exercise should be slow enough for the client to maintain control over the weight. Rapid concentric movement creates too much momentum, so that the muscle is not stimulated during the latter portion of the concentric action. Rapid eccentric movements ("dropping" the weight) deprive the muscle of stimulation during the eccentric phase and can also lead to injury.

▸ **Proper Breathing.** Proper breathing entails avoiding the Valsalva maneuver. Clients often perform a Valsalva maneuver (attempting to exhale against a closed glottis, i.e., "straining") during the concentric phase of the lift. This action significantly elevates arterial blood pressure, potentially damaging blood vessels (e.g., Valsalva retinopathy), and can provoke coronary ischemia in heart patients. If the Valsalva maneuver is held for an extended period of time, arterial blood pressure will fall due to impaired venous return, potentially causing fainting and injury. Teach clients to maintain a normal breathing pattern during the lift, such as by exhaling on exertion.

Spotting Technique

Anyone using free weights should have a trainer or lifting partner serve as a spotter to ensure safety. The principal roles of the spotter are as follows:

- ▸ Ensure that the bar is loaded with equal weight on both sides.
- ▸ Ensure that the lifter uses a balanced grip.
- ▸ Assist the lifter in removing the bar from the rack.
- ▸ Be prepared to assist the lifter if he or she loses balance or is unable to complete a repetition.
- ▸ Assist the lifter in returning the bar to the rack.

It is common to observe spotters assisting lifters with virtually every repetition. This is not proper spotting, as it prevents the lifters from developing the confidence and the motor control to handle the weight on their own. Furthermore, this assistance makes it difficult for you to determine the proper rate of progression for the lifters, as it prevents you from knowing their true ability. An exception occurs with the advanced lifting technique of performing only eccentric, or "negative" repetitions. During negative repetitions, the spotter assists the lifter with each concentric lifting of the weight, and then

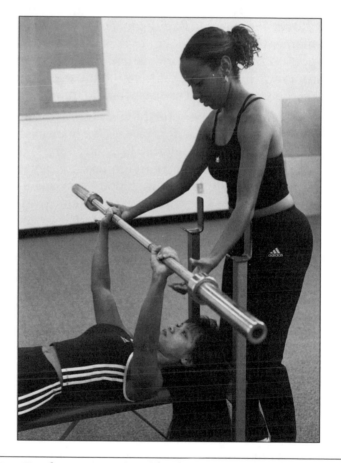

Figure 6.6   Bench press (muscles of the chest—i.e., pectorals; also anterior deltoids, triceps). Lying supine on a bench with the feet planted on the floor for balance, press the weight vertically until the arms are fully extended; then return the weight until the bar touches the chest. The back and buttocks must remain in contact with the bench throughout the lift. The spotter stands behind the lifter's head and bends at the hips and knees, keeping the back in a neutral position, to follow the path of the bar. The spotter's hands are below the bar, in preparation for assisting.

the lifter slowly returns the weight to the starting point. This technique greatly increases delayed-onset muscle soreness and should not be used with novice lifters. Advanced lifters also may use isometric lifts to increase their strength at a particular angle during the repetition. This technique involves overloading the bar, lowering it to the desired angle or "sticking point," and performing an isometric contraction for several seconds. A spotter assists with the placement and removal of the bar.

Figures 6.6-6.14 provide examples of exercises that can be performed using free weights or machines. For a more comprehensive listing of resistance training exercises, see the National Strength and Conditioning Association's 2nd edition of *Essentials of Strength Training and Conditioning* (Baechle and Earle 2000).

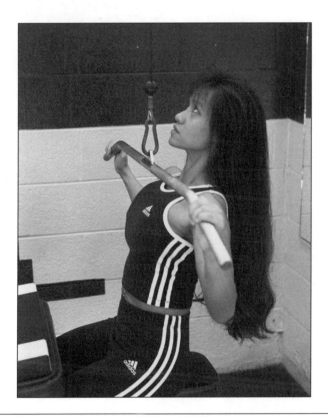

Figure 6.7 Lat pull-down (muscles of the back—i.e., latissimus dorsi; also teres major, biceps). From a seated position and using a widely spaced pronated (overhand) grip, pull the bar down in front of the head until it touches the upper chest; then return the bar to full arm extension.

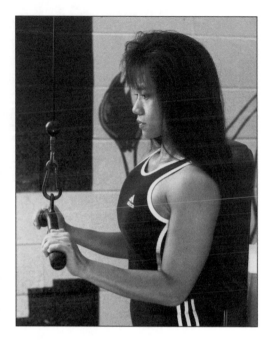

Figure 6.8 Triceps extension (muscles of the posterior upper arm—i.e., triceps). From a standing position with the elbows held against the sides and the forearms approximately 30° above horizontal, press the bar downward to full extension; then return the bar to the starting position. Do not allow the bar to recover to a position higher than 30° above horizontal, which would cause the elbows to swing upward.

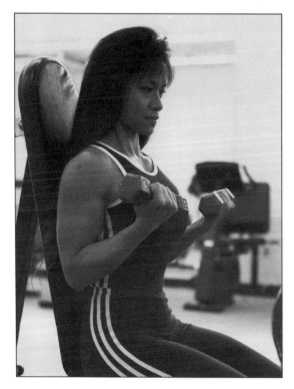

Figure 6.9 Biceps curl (muscles of the anterior upper arm—biceps, brachialis, brachioradialis). From a seated position against back support, and with the elbows held against the sides, lift the dumbbells upward until the elbow is fully flexed; then return the weights to the fully extended position.

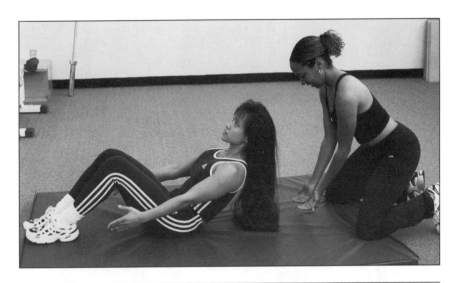

Figure 6.10 Curl-ups (abdominal muscles—rectus abdominis, obliques). Lying supine but with the knees bent 90° and the feet flat on the floor, curl the trunk upward until the shoulder blades are off the floor and the trunk reaches 30° above horizontal. The arms may be held at the side along the floor. A partner may support the head at the end of each repetition to avoid neck strain.

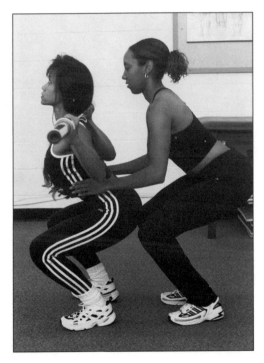

Figure 6.11 Squats (muscles of the thigh and hips—quadriceps, gluteus maximus; also hamstrings, vasti, erector spinae). From a standing position with the feet at least shoulder-width apart and with the bar balanced on the upper back or shoulders, squat down until the thighs are parallel to the floor; then return to the standing position. Keep the head up to help maintain a relatively straight position of the back. Do not curve the back downward, and do not lower the thighs below parallel. The spotter stands behind the lifter and mimics the lifter's movement. The spotter's hands are positioned to lift the torso if needed.

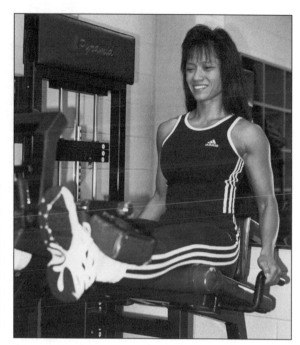

Figure 6.12 Leg extension (muscles of the anterior thigh—quadriceps). From a seated position with the pad adjusted to just above the ankles, lift the weight to full extension of the knees; then return to the starting position.

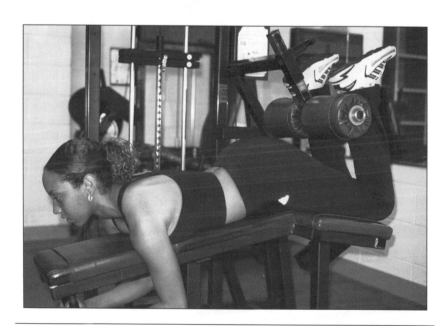

Figure 6.13 Leg curl (muscles of the posterior thigh—hamstrings). Lying face down, slowly pull with your legs until your heels almost touch your gluteal muscles; then return to the starting position.

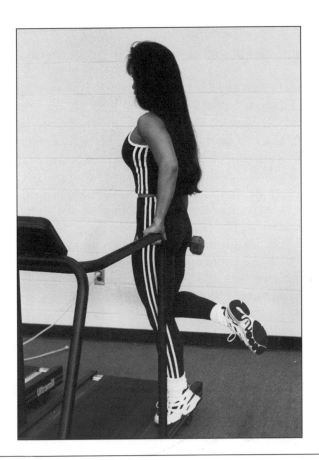

Figure 6.14 Calf raises (muscles of the posterior lower leg—gastrocnemius, soleus). From a standing position with one foot on an elevated surface, one hand holding a support for balance, and one hand holding a dumbbell, rise up on your toes as high as possible, then return to a position below parallel. Standing calf raises emphasize the gastrocnemius muscle, whereas seated calf raises, in which the knee is bent, emphasize the soleus muscle.

CASE STUDY 6.1

Sedentary Client

Tanya G. is a 25-year-old, 145-lb female who is 5'4" tall (BMI of 24.9 kg·m⁻²). She has decided that it is time to "get into shape" and "tone up." Ms. G. has not exercised aerobically since a high school physical education class and has never performed resistance training. She is a former cigarette smoker, having quit three

(continued)

Case Study 6.1 *(continued)*

months ago. She has no signs or symptoms of cardiopulmonary disease.

Ms. G. has two risk factors: sedentary behavior and cigarette smoking (she has to have quit for at least six months before we can discount that risk), placing her in the moderate-risk category. Therefore, she can begin a moderate-intensity exercise program without first seeking physician clearance. In consultation with her, you decide that Ms. G. will exercise three days per week, performing 30 minutes of aerobic work, followed by 30 minutes of flexibility stretching and resistance training, for a total of 60 minutes each session. The first step should be to develop the aerobic workout. You design the program at an intensity that will allow Ms. G. to exercise continually for 30 minutes. The advantages of the aerobic program will be to condition the heart, expend calories, and warm up the muscles in preparation for the second phase, which will be the stretches. You decide to have Ms. G. walk on a treadmill using a target heart rate based on 60-80% of her heart rate reserve. Her estimated maximal HR is $220 - 30 = 190$ bpm. We measure her resting HR as 90 bpm.

$$\text{Target HR} = (\text{intensity fraction})(\text{HRmax} - \text{HRrest}) + \text{HRrest}$$
$$\text{Lower target HR} = (0.6)(190 - 90) + 90$$
$$= (0.6)(100) + 90$$
$$= 60 + 90$$
$$= 150 \text{ bpm}$$
$$\text{Upper target HR} = (0.8)(190 - 90) + 90$$
$$= (0.8)(100) + 90$$
$$= 80 + 90$$
$$= 170 \text{ bpm}$$

You instruct her that, once she has completed her aerobic exercise and is thoroughly warmed up, she should perform the static stretches listed in figures 6.1-6.5 (in that order), holding each for 10-30 seconds, and doing 3-4 sets of the routine.

Ms. G.'s resistance training program will use both free weights and machines. Have her start with the muscles of the upper body and finish with the lower-body muscles. By following the order in figures 6.6-6.14, her first exercises will be compound (those that involve more than one joint, and therefore more than one large muscle or muscle group), and her later exercises will be more isolated (involving only one joint and smaller muscles). To determine the resistance to use, help Ms. G. pick a weight that she can lift comfortably 8-12 times, and increase the weight when she can do 12 repetitions.

CASE STUDY 6.2
Novice Bodybuilder

Carlton B. is a 24-year-old, 220-lb male who wants to compete in his first bodybuilding contest five months from now. Mr. B. has asked your advice on aerobic and weightlifting exercises. His current body fat percentage is 25%. Mr. B. feels that he will probably have to be at about 10% body fat to compete in the bodybuilding competition. Although he feels he is in "pretty good shape," you discover that he performs almost no aerobic exercise for fear that he will lose muscle mass. Mr. B. informs you that he has been lifting weights for five years and feels his muscle and strength gains have plateaued. Mr. B.'s mother had coronary angioplasty at the age of 53, but he has no other risk factors, signs, or symptoms. He has a resting HR of 85 bpm.

Since Mr. B. has only one risk factor (family history) and is young, placing him in the low-risk category, you can confidently proceed with his exercise prescription. Since he has reached a plateau in his training, you prescribe a more advanced routine that involves training specific muscle groups at different times rather than all muscle groups in each workout. Furthermore, because Mr. B. has been lifting weights and is familiar with the amount he is able to lift, it is not necessary to calculate a 1-RM for each weight lifting exercise. You recommend the following resistance training workout, with each exercise preceded by a warm-up set at a relatively light weight:

- ▶ **Frequency:** Twice per week for each routine
- ▶ **Duration:** Three sets each of three to four different exercises (totaling 9-12 sets) for each body part or muscle group
- ▶ **Intensity:** Eight to ten reps per set. When 10 reps are achieved in any one set, increase the weight for that set so that at least

(continued)

Case Study 6.2 *(continued)*

8 reps can be performed. Continue to increase the repetitions to 10 before adding weight.

- ▸ Day 1: Back and biceps exercises
- ▸ Day 2: Legs and abdominals
- ▸ Day 3: Chest and triceps
- ▸ Days 4-6: Repeat days 1-3
- ▸ Day 7: Off

Mr. B.'s goal for body composition is to reach 10% fat. This is still fairly high for a competitive bodybuilder, but is a reasonable goal for his first contest. Determine the amount of fat weight he must lose to accomplish this goal as follows:

$$\text{Goal weight} = \frac{(\text{current weight})(1 - \text{current \%fat})}{(1 - \text{desired \%fat})}$$
$$= (220)(1 - 0.25)/(1 - 0.1)$$
$$= (220)(0.75)/(0.9)$$
$$= 165/0.9$$
$$= 183 \text{ lb}$$

Mr. B. needs to lose 37 lb of fat to reach his goal. Since he has five months to lose this weight, he needs to lose almost 2 lb per week. This gradual weight loss will be important in ensuring that he loses only fat and not muscle. After you reassure Mr. B. that aerobic exercise, if not done in excess, will not reduce his muscle mass, he agrees to follow your recommendations. For the aerobic portion, because Mr. B. has 37 pounds to lose and because he needs to train his cardiovascular system, you recommend that Mr. B. do his aerobic exercise at least four times per week. If he does his aerobic workouts on the same days as the resistance training, he should do the resistance training first, since muscular strength and size are his primary goals. You recommend some light stretching before his resistance training, followed by more aggressive stretching after the completion of the aerobic workout.

You decide to use the heart rate reserve method for Mr. B. and prescribe a target heart rate in the range of 60-85% HRR. His estimated maximal HR is $220 - 24 = 196$ bpm. As reported earlier, his resting HR is 85 bpm.

Target HR = (intensity fraction)(HRmax – HRrest) + HRrest
Lower target HR = (0.6)(196 – 85) + 85
= (0.6)(111) + 85
= 66.6 + 85
= 152 bpm
Upper target HR = (0.85)(196 – 85) + 85
= (0.85)(111) + 85
= 94.35 + 85
= 179 bpm

Next, because Mr. B. must lose 37 pounds, he wants to know how many calories he is expending during his aerobic exercise so he can adjust his food intake. You can calculate this if you know the $\dot{V}O_2$ during his aerobic exercise. Mr. B. informs you that to attain his target heart rate, he must jog on the treadmill at 5 mph up an 8% grade. Use the running equation in table 4.1 to determine his $\dot{V}O_2$. His speed in m·min^{-1} is (5 mph) × 26.8 = 134 m·min^{-1}.

$\dot{V}O_2$ = 3.5 + 0.2(speed) + 0.9(speed)(fractional grade)
= 3.5 + 0.2(134) + 0.9(134)(0.08)
= 3.5 + 26.8 + 9.6
= 39.9 ml·min^{-1}·kg^{-1} (gross $\dot{V}O_2$)
net $\dot{V}O_2$ = 39.9 – 3.5 = 36.4 ml·min^{-1}·kg^{-1}

Now that you have calculated Mr. B.'s $\dot{V}O_2$, you can determine the number of calories he burns during a 30-minute aerobic session. Remember to subtract the resting energy expenditure, or 1 MET (3.5 ml·min^{-1}·kg^{-1}), and report *net* calories burned. To calculate net calories burned, first convert the answer to liters per minute for his entire weight, in this case 100 kg:

(36.4 ml·min^{-1}·kg^{-1})(100 kg)/1000 = 3.64 L·min^{-1}

Since 5 kilocalories are expended for each liter of oxygen consumed, during a 30-minute exercise session Mr. B. would burn the following number of calories:

(3.64 L·min^{-1}) × (5 kcal·L^{-1}) = 18.2 kcal·min^{-1}
(18.2 kcal·min^{-1}) × (30 min) = 546 kcal per session

(continued)

Case Study 6.2   *(continued)*

Note that 546 kcal are much more than the average individual normally burns during 30 minutes of exercise. But Mr. B. is a large person, in fairly good condition. Since he is performing this exercise four times per week, his total caloric expenditure from aerobic exercise is 546 × 4 = 2184 kcal per week. This represents 2184 / 3500 = 0.6 lb of fat. Although his weight training is also greater than it was before, he still needs to adjust his diet to achieve his target of losing nearly 2 lb of fat per week, especially avoiding fatty foods.

REFERENCES

1. Baechle, TR, and RW Earle, eds. 2000. *Essentials of Strength Training and Conditioning*, 2nd ed. Champaign, IL: Human Kinetics.
2. Franklin, BA, ed. 2000. *ACSM's Guidelines for Exercise Testing and Prescription*, 6th ed., 156-160. Philadelphia: Lippincott Williams & Wilkins.
3. Pollock, ML, GA Gaesser, JD Butcher, JP Despres, RK Dishman, BA Franklin, and CE Garber. 1998. The recommended quantity and quality of exercise for developing and maintaining cardiorespiratory and muscular fitness, and flexibility in healthy adults (ACSM position stand). *Med. Sci. Sports Exerc.* 30:975-991.

7

Exercise Prescription for the Older Adult

Aging is associated with a decline in physical function and, in many cases, a loss of independence. But is aging itself the root cause of these changes? Certainly, some physical decline can be expected as a biological consequence of age, but much of what is called aging is simply the result of years of physical inactivity. Those who remain physically active throughout life demonstrate much slower rates of physical decline than do the sedentary. And a growing body of research indicates that those who have been sedentary for many years can experience significant improvements by beginning an exercise program even at very advanced ages.

As table 7.1 summarizes, properly prescribed exercise for elderly people can significantly improve their aerobic power (Ehsani 1987), muscular strength and size (Fiatarone et al. 1990; Fiatarone et al. 1994; Frontera et al. 1988), and bone density (Dalsky 1989; Menkes et al. 1993). Improvements in functional measures such as walking speed and stair-climbing power have also been reported (Fiatarone et al. 1990; Fiatarone et al. 1994). These results can reverse the effects of many years of physical decline, and lead to greater independence and a much higher quality of life.

Table 7.1

Adaptations in the Elderly to Exercise Training

- ► Increased aerobic power, $\dot{V}O_2$max
- ► Increased lactate threshold
- ► Increased muscular strength, 1-RM
- ► Increased muscle cross-sectional area
- ► Increased bone mineral density
- ► Increased walking speed
- ► Increased stair-climbing power

The principles of exercise prescription described in preceding chapters apply to the elderly as well as to younger adults. You may need to modify the guidelines somewhat based on initial fitness level, orthopedic problems, complicating medical conditions, and the effects of medications. Making allowance for these issues *on an individual basis* is the key to adapting the general principles to the elderly.

Do not make the mistake of assuming that all elderly are of a low fitness level. The range of individual variability among the elderly is very large. Whereas some older people are frail and need assistance to accomplish activities of daily living (ADL), others are highly fit and enjoy challenging themselves physically. Many individuals in their 60s, 70s, and beyond run marathons, participate in century (100-mile) bike rides, do competitive powerlifting, and go on multiday backpacking treks.

The ACSM's *Guidelines* provide specific recommendations for writing exercise prescriptions for the elderly (Franklin 2000). Although the ACSM offers no special changes from the standard recommendations for flexibility training in the elderly, it does prescribe modifications for cardiovascular fitness and resistance training.

CARDIOVASCULAR FITNESS

Since many elderly have a low initial fitness level, it is prudent to begin exercise prescriptions at a low intensity and to progress gradually. However, the intensity range of 40/50% to 85% of $\dot{V}O_2R$ still applies—just make more frequent use of the low end of this range for initial prescriptions with the elderly.

When prescribing exercise intensity by heart rate, you must consider several factors. Remember that, for adults of any age, formulas for estimating maximal heart rate (such as 220 – age) provide only rough approximations. This is especially true for older adults, as the range of actual maximal heart rates grows larger with age. Thus, you should use great caution in applying target HR ranges with elderly clients unless the ranges are based on *measured* maximum heart rates.

Chapter 3 stated that the %HRR method is superior to the %HRmax method for establishing target heart rates. For the elderly, the ACSM notes that the %HRmax method is better than the %HRR method for indicating a given level of %$\dot{V}O_2$max. This would be true for anyone of a low fitness level, regardless of age; but it is misleading in regard to exercise prescriptions. As chapter 2 discussed, we now prescribe exercise intensity as a percentage of $\dot{V}O_2$ *reserve*, not as a percentage of $\dot{V}O_2$*max*. Percentage of HRR provides equivalent exercise intensities to %$\dot{V}O_2R$ for older as well as younger adults. A further argument giving preference to the %HRR method is that many elderly have elevated resting heart rates, which causes problems when target heart rates are prescribed by %HRmax. As an example in chapter 3 illustrates, the use of %HRmax for elderly clients sometimes results in target heart rates that are little more than resting heart rate. *For these reasons, the authors recommend %HRR as the preferred method of prescribing target heart rates in the elderly, just as with younger adults.*

The mode of exercise is an important consideration with the elderly, since the best program for counteracting osteoporosis may increase orthopedic problems. To reduce orthopedic stress, minimize weightbearing activities—aquatic exercise is a very good choice. To combat osteoporosis and improve bone density, however, you must maximize weightbearing activities—which means aquatic exercise would be a poor choice. The solution to this dilemma is to individualize every program, prescribing weightbearing exercise *within the client's orthopedic tolerance level.* Walking is an excellent choice for many older people.

Other considerations regarding the mode of exercise: use group exercise as much as possible to engender compliance through social support; when choosing aerobic machines, avoid those with excessively complicated panels and programs.

RESISTANCE TRAINING

The ACSM's recommendations for the elderly differ significantly from its standard recommendations for resistance training. As described below, and summarized in table 7.2, the present authors take issue with three of these points.

Table 7.2

Differences in ACSM's and Authors' Recommendations for Exercise Prescriptions for the Elderly

Issue	ACSM	Authors
HR prescription	Use %HRmax	Use %HRR
Resistance training intensity	RPE of 12-13	8-12 RM
Initial adaptation period for resistance training	8 weeks at minimal resistance	1-2 weeks at minimal resistance
Equipment for resistance training	Machines preferred over free weights	Free weights stress balance and have smaller weight increments

---

The ACSM sets the intensity level for the elderly at 10-15 repetitions at a perceived exertion of 12-13 ("somewhat hard"), vs. an intensity at the 8-12 RM for younger adults. Lifting to the point of failure in 8 to 12 repetitions requires much more effort than performing 10 to 15 repetitions at a level that seems somewhat hard. This is a curious recommendation from the ACSM for two reasons. First, the RPE scale is not generally used for gauging intensity during weightlifting. Second, research with elderly subjects (including nonagenarians) has established that large improvements in strength and modest, yet statistically significant, improvements in muscle size are achieved with sets performed for 8 repetitions at 80% of 1-RM (Fiatarone et al. 1990; Fiatarone et al. 1994; Frontera et al. 1988). For most resistance exercises, a weight set at 80% of 1-RM can be lifted approximately 10 times. Thus, it would appear that the elderly should use the same 8-12 repetition range to failure that is recommended by the ACSM for younger clients. Elderly clients may be using a low absolute intensity (i.e., a low weight), but should not be using a low relative intensity (i.e., % of 1-RM).

Clients should choose a weight that they can lift eight times, and attempt to perform additional repetitions during succeeding exercise sessions. Once the client is able to lift the weight 12 times, the weight should be increased for the following session. The increase should be small (approximately 10%), and designed to bring the client back to the 8-RM level.

Another questionable recommendation by the ACSM is that the elderly should use minimal resistance for the first eight weeks of a program. The training studies cited earlier used only one week of familiarization before setting the resistance at 80% of 1-RM (Fiatarone et al. 1990; Fiatarone et al. 1994; Frontera et al. 1988). One of the authors of this book (DPS) has considerable experience in resistance training with the elderly, and uses a one- to two-week period for initial adjustment to the program. This period of time is important for teaching proper lifting technique and for minimizing **delayed-onset muscle soreness (DOMS).** Clients who have not performed resistance exercise for several decades, if ever, must be cautioned to use very light weights on the first day and to still expect DOMS the following day. It is not necessary to attempt 1-RM lifts initially, or to find the 8-RM by trial and error on the first day of training. Rather, *the weight chosen for the first few sessions should feel easy throughout a set of 12 or 15 repetitions.* The last repetition need not be challenging. Once you are satisfied that the client is using proper form, which should take no longer than two weeks, you can determine the 8-RM by trial and error, using that figure to establish the intensity for the progressive phase of training.

A third ACSM recommendation for the elderly that bears some scrutiny is the recommendation to use machines as opposed to free weights. It is true that machines require less skill, but free weights have the advantage of teaching balance and greater neuromuscular control, which may be transferrable to real-world activities. Furthermore, free weights are superior for providing small increments of weight. Most exercises can be performed with dumbbells or ankle weights, which come in 1-pound (0.45 kg) increments at the low end, and 5-pound (2.3 kg) increments at the high end. A significant disadvantage of machines is that the increments are usually 10 pounds (4.5 kg) or more. A client performing 12 repetitions with 20 pounds (9.1 kg) on a machine is faced with the daunting prospect of moving up to 30 pounds (13.6 kg), a 50% increase! Fortunately, this can be remedied by attaching a 1- or 2-pound (0.45 or 0.9 kg) free weight to the machine's weight stack.

The ACSM offers these important recommendations for elderly resistance trainers: do not exercise during an acute arthritic flare-up; exercise only within a pain-free range of motion; and reduce the load by 50% or more when returning from a layoff. In all other aspects of resistance training, the ACSM's recommendations for the elderly are the same as for younger adults.

CASE STUDY 7.1
Older Adult With Low Initial Fitness

Bart B. is 82 years old. He is 6'1" tall and weighs 182 lbs. His total cholesterol is 218 $mg \cdot dl^{-1}$, LDL is 120 $mg \cdot dl^{-1}$, HDL is 43 $mg \cdot dl^{-1}$, and fasting glucose is 101 $mg \cdot dl^{-1}$. He has no family or personal history of heart disease. He has arthritis in his hands and knees, which usually does not prevent him from carrying out activities of daily living. He quit smoking 20 years ago. His blood pressure is 146/86 mmHg, with resting HR of 84 bpm. He plays golf infrequently. He reports no signs or symptoms of cardiopulmonary disease. He has recently undergone a fitness evaluation with the following results: 18 $ml \cdot min^{-1} \cdot kg^{-1}$ estimated $\dot{V}O_2max$ from a submaximal bike test; he can do three push-ups, no partial (Canadian) curl-ups, and achieved 23 cm as his sit-and-reach score (on a 26 cm foot-line box). Stratify Mr. B.'s risk and assess his fitness. Design a comprehensive exercise prescription for him.

Mr. B. has two risk factors: hypertension and sedentary lifestyle. His BMI is 24 $kg \cdot m^{-2}$, well below the criterion for risk (which is 30 $kg \cdot m^{-2}$). His total cholesterol is elevated, but is not a risk factor because his LDL is below the threshold of 130 $mg \cdot dl^{-1}$. His age and his two risk factors place Mr. B. in the moderate-risk category. It would be prudent for him to see his physician concerning his desire to exercise, but it is reasonable for him to begin a moderate exercise program at this time. Mr. B.'s arthritis is manageable, but will need to be considered during his exercise training.

Mr. B.'s body composition appears to be normal, although this is based only on BMI. Based on normative tables from chapter 4 of ACSM's sixth edition *Guidelines* (Franklin 2000), most of his fitness levels are well below average. Note, however, that the oldest age range for the ACSM norms is 60+ years, and may not provide an accurate representation of octogenarians in the population. His aerobic capacity of 18 ml·min^{-1}·kg^{-1} is below the 10th percentile. His muscular strength/endurance is also very low, as three push-ups place him at about the 15th percentile; and he was unable to perform a single partial curl-up with good form. His sit-and-reach score of 23 cm means that he is not quite able to reach his toes (at the 26-cm mark) and places him at about the 55th percentile. Appropriate goals for Mr. B. at this time would be to improve his aerobic capacity and muscular strength to the average level for 60+ year old males, and to maintain or improve his flexibility.

Follow the general guidelines in table 2.1 for Mr. B's exercise prescription. You begin his cardiovascular conditioning at three sessions per week on alternate days, for 20 minutes per session, at an intensity approximating 40-60% of $\dot{V}O_2R$. Given his low initial fitness level, his manageable level of arthritis, and your desire to incorporate weightbearing activity into his program, you recommend walking as the principal mode of exercise. You should monitor his arthritis symptoms and ask him to back off if they worsen. The simplest way to assign Mr. B. to an intensity of 40-60% $\dot{V}O_2R$ may be to use the talk test, or an RPE of 12-14 (from table 3.1). Alternatively, you could calculate a target heart rate based on 64-77% of HRmax (from table 3.1) or based on 40-60% of HRR. These values are 88-106 bpm using %HRmax, and 106-116 bpm using %HRR (see below for the calculations). Given his resting HR of 84 bpm, the values derived from %HRmax would appear to be too low. In either case, since these target HRs were calculated using an estimated HRmax of 220 – age, you understand that they are very rough estimates.

%HRmax method:

$$\text{Lower target HR} = 0.64(220 - 82)$$
$$= 0.64(138)$$
$$= 88 \text{ bpm}$$
$$\text{Upper target HR} = 0.77(138)$$
$$= 106 \text{ bpm}$$

(continued)

Case Study 7.1   *(continued)*

%HRR method:

Target HR = (intensity fraction)(HRmax − HRrest) + HRrest

$$\text{Lower target HR} = 0.40(138 − 84) + 84$$
$$= 0.40(54) + 84$$
$$= 22 + 84$$
$$= 106 \text{ bpm}$$
$$\text{Upper target HR} = 0.60(138 − 84) + 84$$
$$= 0.60(54) + 84$$
$$= 32 + 84$$
$$= 116 \text{ bpm}$$

Another means of setting the intensity would be to calculate a walking speed at 40-60% of $\dot{V}O_2R$. Using the walking equation from table 4.1, this would be 2.2-3.2 mph (see below for calculations). This also is only a rough estimate of the exercise intensity, because it is based on an estimated $\dot{V}O_2$max, which furthermore was an estimate made during cycling exercise rather than during walking.

Target $\dot{V}O_2$= (intensity fraction)($\dot{V}O_2$max − 3.5) + 3.5

$$\text{Lower target } \dot{V}O_2 = 0.40(18 − 3.5) + 3.5$$
$$= 0.40(14.5) + 3.5$$
$$= 5.8 + 3.5$$
$$= 9.3 \text{ ml·min}^{-1}\text{·kg}^{-1}$$
$$\text{Upper target } \dot{V}O_2 = 0.60(18 − 3.5) + 3.5$$
$$= 0.60(14.5) + 3.5$$
$$= 8.7 + 3.5$$
$$= 12.2 \text{ ml·min}^{-1}\text{·kg}^{-1}$$

Now, calculate the desired walking speed using the walking equation from table 4.1.

$\dot{V}O_2$ = 3.5 + 0.1(speed) + 1.8(speed)(fractional grade)

Lower target workload:

$$9.3 = 3.5 + 0.1(\text{speed}) + 1.8(\text{speed})(0)$$
$$9.3 = 3.5 + 0.1(\text{speed})$$

$$9.3 - 3.5 = 0.1(\text{speed})$$
$$5.8 = 0.1(\text{speed})$$
$$5.8/0.1 = \text{speed}$$
$$58 \text{ m·min}^{-1} = \text{speed}$$
$$(58 \text{ m·min}^{-1})/26.8 = 2.2 \text{ mph}$$

Upper target workload:

$$12.2 = 3.5 + 0.1(\text{speed})$$
$$12.2 - 3.5 = 0.1(\text{speed})$$
$$8.7 = 0.1(\text{speed})$$
$$8.7/0.1 = \text{speed}$$
$$87 \text{ m·min}^{-1} = \text{speed}$$
$$(87 \text{ m·min}^{-1})/26.8 = 3.2 \text{ mph}$$

To summarize, you can estimate the intensity as a HR or walking speed, but you must closely observe Mr. B.'s responses to the exercise to determine if he appears to be exercising at a light to moderate level. If he has difficulty completing 20 minutes at this level, you need to reduce the intensity. If he finds that 20 minutes at this level is very easy, increase the intensity until it feels somewhat hard. Once you have established the proper intensity, Mr. B. can enter the improvement phase, in which he gradually increases the duration and frequency of his cardiovascular exercise. Furthermore, as his ability improves, he can increase his absolute intensity (i.e., walking speed) while leaving his relative intensity (i.e., HR) within the target range.

Mr. B. should perform his resistance training program two or three times per week. If he is exercising in your facility three times per week for cardiovascular conditioning, it might be useful to have him perform his resistance training as part of the same sessions. Teach him how to properly perform a variety of exercises that target all of the major muscle groups. Pay special attention to lifting technique, range of motion through a pain-free arc, proper breathing (avoiding the Valsalva maneuver), and a controlled speed of movement through both the concentric (lifting) and eccentric (lowering) phases. He should begin with very light weights while learning proper technique. Once he has developed skill at the various lifts and has overcome his initial soreness, assist Mr. B. in selecting

(continued)

Case Study 7.1   *(continued)*

weights that provide the appropriate intensity for the improvement phase of the program—10-15 "somewhat hard" repetitions in accordance with ACSM guidelines, or 8-12 repetitions to volitional fatigue if you follow the present authors' recommendations. He should perform at least one set of each of the selected exercises. A preferred routine might be to perform one set at 50% of the prescribed intensity as a warm-up, and then one or two sets at the prescribed intensity. The routine should allow completion of all lifts in no more than one hour, and preferably in 20-30 minutes.

Mr. B. does not need to place a lot of emphasis on the flexibility aspect of his training program, at least with regard to his measured lower back and hamstring flexibility. However, to insure maintenance of good all-round flexibility, at the conclusion of each exercise session he should perform a variety of flexibility exercises targeting all major muscle groups. These exercises should follow the general guidelines summarized in table 2.1, in which each stretch is taken to a position of mild discomfort and held for 10-30 seconds. He should perform each stretch three or four times.

CASE STUDY 7.2
Older Adult With High Initial Fitness

Francine A. is 66 years old. She is 5'5" tall, and weighs 136 lb. A long-distance cyclist who has ridden across several states, she averages 10-15 hours of bicycling per week. Her total cholesterol is 193 mg·dl^{-1}, LDL is 102 mg·dl^{-1}, HDL is 64 mg·dl^{-1}, and fasting glucose is 88 mg·dl^{-1}. Her father had a heart attack at 53 years of age. She is a nonsmoker. Her blood pressure is 118/74 mmHg, and her resting HR is 62 bpm. She reports no signs or symptoms of cardiopulmonary disease. A recent fitness evaluation yielded the following results: 44 ml·min^{-1}·kg^{-1} estimated $\dot{V}O_2$max from a submaximal bike test, 45 lb for a 1-RM bench press, 170 lb for a 1-RM leg press, 10 modified push-ups, 3 partial (Canadian) curl-ups, and 21 cm sit-and-reach score (on a 26 cm foot-line box). Stratify Ms. A.'s risk and assess her fitness. Design a comprehensive exercise prescription for her.

Ms. A. has only one risk factor: family history. However, because she has the negative risk factor of a high HDL level (above 60 mg·dl^{-1}), we would count her as having zero risk factors for screening purposes. Nevertheless, Ms. A. is in the moderate-risk category because of her age. You can safely place her in a moderate-intensity exercise program.

Ms. A.'s body composition is considered normal, based on a BMI of 23 $kg \cdot m^{-2}$. Her aerobic capacity of 44 $ml \cdot min^{-1} \cdot kg^{-1}$ is excellent for her age group, being in the 90th percentile based on the table of norms in chapter 4 of the sixth edition of the ACSM's *Guidelines* (Franklin 2000). Her muscular fitness presents a mixed picture. You can evaluate her upper-body strength from her bench press 1-RM, expressed as a fraction of her body weight (45/136 = 0.33). This value places her in the 10th percentile. Her lower-body strength is much better, as her 1-RM/body weight ratio for the leg press is 1.25, placing her at approximately the 85th percentile. Her upper-body muscular endurance is better than her upper body strength, since her 10 modified push-ups is at the 60th percentile. Her abdominal muscle endurance is not as good, with three partial curl-ups at the 30th percentile. Finally, the flexibility of her lower back and hamstrings, as indicated by a sit-and-reach score of 21 cm, places her at about the 15th percentile. In summary, although Ms. A. has very good aerobic capacity and leg strength from her bicycling, she needs to improve in other areas. Goals for Ms. A. would be to maintain her aerobic capacity and leg strength, and to improve to at least the average level in her muscular strength, muscular endurance, and flexibility.

Ms. A. does not need any guidance regarding her cardiovascular conditioning. If she wants a target range, you could suggest 60-80% of $\dot{V}O_2R$. From table 3.1, you could estimate this intensity as 77-91% of HRmax, or 119-140 bpm; or, using 60-80% of HRR, her target HRs would be 117-136 bpm (see below for calculations). Note that, since she has a low resting HR, the %HRmax and %HRR methods yield similar answers. However, you should use caution in applying these values, as they were calculated with HRmax estimated as 220 – age.

%HRmax method:

$$\text{Lower target HR} = 0.77(220 - 66)$$
$$= 0.77(154)$$
$$= 119 \text{ bpm}$$
$$\text{Upper target HR} = 0.91(154)$$
$$= 140 \text{ bpm}$$

(continued)

Case Study 7.2 *(continued)*

%HRR method:

Target HR = (intensity fraction)(HRmax − HRrest) + HRrest

$$\text{Lower target HR} = 0.60(154 - 62) + 62$$
$$= 0.60(92) + 62$$
$$= 55 + 62$$
$$= 117 \text{ bpm}$$
$$\text{Upper target HR} = 0.80(154 - 62) + 62$$
$$= 0.80(92) + 62$$
$$= 74 + 62$$
$$= 136 \text{ bpm}$$

Ms. A. would definitely benefit from a resistance training program. Given her excellent leg strength, she should emphasize upper-body and trunk exercises. However, she also should include leg exercises in order to balance her development. As with Mr. B. above, she should perform her resistance training program two to three days per week, using at least one set of each exercise performed at a "somewhat hard" level for 10-15 repetitions (to follow ACSM guidelines), or at the 8-12 RM (to follow recommendations of the authors).

Ms. A. should follow a well-designed flexibility program that includes a variety of stretches that target all major muscle groups (with special attention to her low back and hamstring area, which needs improvement), performed for three to four repetitions of 10-30 seconds, each at a position of mild discomfort. Rather than limiting herself to doing these exercises after her resistance training two to three times per week, she also should stretch after her aerobic workouts, which she does on an almost daily basis.

REFERENCES

1. Dalsky, GP. 1989. The role of exercise in the prevention of osteoporosis. *Compr. Ther.* 15(9):30-37.

2. Ehsani, AA. 1987. Cardiovascular adaptations to exercise training in the elderly. *Fed. Proc.* 46:1840-1843.

3. Fiatarone, MA, EC Marks, ND Ryan, CN Meredith, LA Lipsitz, and WJ Evans. 1990. High intensity strength training in nonagenarians. *J. Am. Med. Assoc.* 263:3029-3034.

4. Fiatarone, MA, EF O'Neill, ND Ryan, KM Clements, GR Solares, ME Nelson, SB Roberts, JJ Kehayias, LA Lipsitz, and WJ Evans. 1994. Exercise training and nutritional supplementation for physical frailty in very elderly people. *New Eng. J. Med.* 330:1769-1775.

5. Franklin, BA, ed. 2000. *ACSM's Guidelines for Exercise Testing and Prescription*, 6th ed., 67-88, 223-230. Philadelphia: Lippincott Williams & Wilkins.

6. Frontera, WR, CN Meredith, KP O'Reilly, HG Knuttgen, and WJ Evans. 1988. Strength conditioning in older men: skeletal muscle hypertrophy and improved function. *J. Appl. Physiol.* 64:1038-1044.

7. Menkes, A, S Mazel, RA Redmond, K Koffler, CR Libinati, CM Gundberg, TM Zizic, JM Hagberg, RE Pratley, and BF Hurley. 1993. Strength training increases regional bone mineral density and bone remodeling in middle-aged and older men. *J. Appl. Physiol.* 74:2478-2484.

CHAPTER

8

Exercise Prescription for Heart Disease

Heart disease, or **coronary artery disease,** is the number one cause of death in the United States. When a person exercises, the heart must work harder and its demand for blood flow and oxygen increases. A person with clinically significant coronary heart disease cannot increase the flow of blood and oxygen to the heart sufficiently during such times of increased demand, which can result in chest pain, or **angina.** Angina may result when a coronary artery is blocked 50% or more, as seen on an angiographic view of the artery during a heart catheterization (Wenger and Hellerstein 1992). Most people do not notice heart disease resulting from atherosclerosis, or blocked arteries, until they experience significant symptoms or damage. Other types of heart disease may result from valve damage and high blood pressure. **Myocardial infarctions (MIs)** can cause extensive damage to the heart that can result in congestive heart failure. Some patients may even require pacemakers or automatic defibrillators for the management of **arrhythmias.**

EXERCISE FOR HEART DISEASE

Exercise benefits people with heart disease in many ways. Regular exercise decreases sympathetic drive, which reduces both blood pressure and heart rate during submaximal exercise and at rest. This means that the patient can perform a given amount of work with less demand (a lower rate × pressure product) on the heart. Reduced sympathetic drive also decreases ventricular irritability, which can diminish the risk of serious arrhythmias. Regular exercise also reduces the risk for further progression of heart disease, by reducing LDL cholesterol, increasing HDL cholesterol, reducing obesity, and reducing sympathetically mediated blood pressure and platelet stickiness. One study that incorporated regular exercise with a low-fat diet and stress reduction found that such a comprehensive plan resulted in actual regression of coronary blockage (Ornish et al. 1990). In that study, the subjects who performed the most exercise, averaging an hour a day at a moderate intensity, achieved the best results. Other benefits of exercise for heart disease patients include a reduction in health care costs, a faster return to daily activities after hospitalization, and improvements in functional capacity and self-esteem.

FOUR VARIABLES OF THE FITT PRINCIPLE

Aerobic exercise prescriptions for patients with heart disease should include the four basic variables of the FITT principle: Frequency, Intensity, Time (duration), and Type (mode). Weightlifting also may be added once a regular program of aerobic exercise has been established. You must modify the basic guidelines for exercise prescription according to the individual's clinical status and the phase of rehabilitation.

Standard cardiac rehabilitation programs have four phases. Phase I (inpatient) is usually short in duration (three to five days) and involves patient care in the hospital under the direct supervision of a physician and either a nurse, exercise specialist, or physical therapist. Phase II (outpatient) follows hospital discharge and requires the patient to return to the hospital for rehabilitation, usually lasting 12 weeks. However, many phase II programs now stratify patients according to risk status. According to this stratification or insurance coverage, low-, moderate-, and high-risk patients may train for 6, 8, or 12 weeks, respectively. This phase includes ECG and blood pressure monitoring for most patients, and education. Phase III (community-initial) and Phase IV (community-maintenance) are usually held at a university, health club, or other fitness setting. They are variable in length and include little supervision and monitoring. To be admitted to phase III or IV programs, patients must be clinically stable, have normal blood pressure and ECG responses to exercise, and should have a functional capacity of least 8 METs (Franklin 2000). Patients engaging in inpatient, outpatient, or community exercise should be risk-stratified according to medical history, clinical status, and symptoms.

The exercise prescription during phase I depends strongly on the clinical status of the patient. According to the FITT principle, here is a general exercise prescription for most *inpatients:*

- ▸ **Frequency:** Some type of mobilization at least twice a day (three to four times per day initially) to prevent stasis and clotting of blood
- ▸ **Intensity:** An RPE less than 13, or target heart rate that is 20 bpm above the standing resting HR for post-MI patients (not to exceed 120 bpm), or 30 bpm above standing resting HR for postsurgery patients
- ▸ **Time:** Intermittent bouts lasting three to five minutes, with rest periods shorter than the mobilization time (as tolerated by the patient)—for a total time of 20 minutes
- ▸ **Type:** Mobilization activities such as sitting up in bed with or without assistance, self-care activities, walking in the halls of the hospital, or stationary cycle activity

Exercise prescription for patients involved in phases II-IV are also contingent on clinical status but emphasize education and activities designed to help them return to their premorbid lifestyle. A general exercise prescription for most *outpatients* that follows the FITT principle is as follows:

- ▸ **Frequency:** A minimum of two to three days per week appears to be effective for cardiorespiratory conditioning.
- ▸ **Intensity:** The full range of 40-85% of oxygen uptake reserve ($\dot{V}O_2R$) may be employed; most prescriptions focus on the lower end of this range, depending on patient status. Variables such as ST-segment depression, angina, threatening arrhythmias, and diminished ejection fraction are some of the major factors used to determine patient status or risk (Franklin 2000).

▸ **Time:** To achieve a training effect, 20-60 minutes of continuous or intermittent exercise is required. Patients should progress toward a minimum goal of 1000 kcal per week over a 3-6 month period.

▸ **Type:** Both aerobic and resistance training are utilized. A variety of equipment is recommended—treadmills, cycle and arm ergometers, steppers, rowers, and weight machines. Phases III/IV may include skilled games such as basketball and volleyball.

MYOCARDIAL INFARCTION

A few decades ago, individuals who experienced a heart attack were placed on bed rest for several weeks. Today it is well recognized that bed rest worsens the patient's condition and that early mobilization followed by exercise training is an important means of restoring activities of daily living, improving fitness, and reducing risk factors for the further progression of the disease.

CASE STUDY 8.1
Myocardial Infarction Patient

A 44-year-old, 179-lb corporate executive, Samir H. was admitted to the hospital complaining of chest pain. After evaluation by a cardiologist, it was determined that Mr. H. was experiencing a mild heart attack. He was immediately taken to the catheterization lab where he was diagnosed with a significantly blocked left circumflex artery. Percutaneous coronary angioplasty (PTCA) was performed. A follow-up echocardiography test reported an ejection fraction of 55%, indicating that Mr. H. had not suffered major heart damage. Two weeks later, Mr. H. was referred to you for an exercise prescription in a phase II cardiac rehabilitation program. His only medication is daily aspirin. A maximal treadmill exercise test taking Mr. H. to volitional fatigue after his PTCA revealed the following information:

▸ **ECG:** normal sinus rhythm
▸ **Maximum heart rate:** 156 bpm
▸ **Resting heart rate:** 62 bpm
▸ **Peak blood pressure:** 150/90 mmHg
▸ **Resting blood pressure:** 120/70 mmHg

Because Mr. H.'s heart did not sustain a large amount of damage, and because of his younger age and desire to exercise, you choose a fairly moderate to vigorous window for his intensity, such as 60-80% of $\dot{V}O_2R$ using the %HRR method. He will work up to 45 minutes of this exercise during his phase II sessions, which will be held three times per week.

$$\text{Target HR} = (\text{intensity fraction})(\text{HRmax} - \text{HRrest}) + \text{HRrest}$$
$$\text{Lower target HR} = (0.60)(156 - 62) + 62$$
$$= (0.60)(94) + 62$$
$$= 56 + 62$$
$$= 118 \text{ bpm}$$
$$\text{Upper target HR} = (0.80)(156 - 62) + 62$$
$$= (0.80)(94) + 62$$
$$= 75 + 62$$
$$= 137 \text{ bpm}$$

If Mr. H. performs the exercise as prescribed, will he reach the goal of expending at least 1000 kcal per week? Mr. H. tells you that in order to exercise in his target heart rate range, he must jog on a treadmill at 4 mph, 3% grade. To calculate the $\dot{V}O_2$ for Mr. H., use the running equation from table 4.1. His running speed in $m \cdot min^{-1}$ is (4 mph) $\times$ 26.8 = 107.2 $m \cdot min^{-1}$.

$$\dot{V}O_2 = 3.5 + 0.2(\text{speed}) + 0.9(\text{speed})(\text{fractional grade})$$
$$= 3.5 + 0.2(107.2) + 0.9(107.2)(0.03)$$
$$= 3.5 + 21.4 + 2.9$$
$$= 27.8 \text{ ml} \cdot min^{-1} \cdot kg^{-1} \text{ (gross } \dot{V}O_2)$$
$$\text{Net } \dot{V}O_2 = 27.8 - 3.5 = 24.3 \text{ ml} \cdot min^{-1} \cdot kg^{-1}$$

To calculate *net* calories burned, first convert the answer to liters per minute. Mr. H.'s body mass is (179 lb)/2.2 = 81.4 kg.

$$(24.3 \text{ ml} \cdot min^{-1} \cdot kg^{-1}) \times (81.4 \text{ kg})/1000 = 1.98 \text{ L} \cdot min^{-1}$$

Because 5 kilocalories are expended for each liter of oxygen consumed, Mr. W. would burn the following number of calories:

$$(1.98 \text{ L} \cdot min^{-1}) \times (5 \text{ kcal} \cdot L^{-1}) = 9.9 \text{ kcal} \cdot min^{-1}$$
$$(9.9 \text{ kcal} \cdot min^{-1}) \times (45 \text{ minutes}) = 445 \text{ kcal per exercise session}$$

(continued)

Case Study 8.1   *(continued)*

Phase II meets three times per week, so Mr. H. would burn $445 \times 3 = 1338$ kcal, exceeding the minimum recommended weekly caloric expenditure.

HEART FAILURE

Individuals who suffer significant left ventricular damage after a myocardial infarction will have diminished cardiac output that may progressively worsen and result in peripheral and pulmonary edema. Ejection fractions less than 50% at rest indicate a moderate risk, whereas ejection fractions less than 40% indicate a high risk of developing **congestive heart failure (CHF)**. Nonetheless, individuals with CHF respond positively to an exercise training program.

CASE STUDY 8.2
Congestive Heart Failure Patient

Phillip E. is a 65-year-old retired salesman with a 20-year history of heart disease that includes two myocardial infarctions, each followed by a bypass operation. The most recent bypass was last year. He has decided to begin an exercise program, but because he is experiencing shortness of breath, Mr. E. has wisely decided to seek the recommendation of his physician. The physician ordered a cardiopulmonary exercise stress test and an echocardiography test to evaluate Mr. E.'s heart and exercise capacity. The exercise stress test was performed on a treadmill, using the Modified Bruce protocol, and was terminated at volitional exhaustion. Although Mr. E. reported no cardiac symptoms during the exercise stress test, he had to end the test after just five minutes due to shortness of breath. His echocardiography test reported a low ejection fraction, about 30%. His physician determined that Mr. E. was in congestive heart failure, and he prescribed a diuretic, an ACE inhibitor, and a K^+ supplement. His physician cleared Mr. E. for exercise and referred him to you. The results of the cardiopulmonary exercise stress test were as follows:

- ▸ **ECG:** old myocardial infarctions (significant Q-wave present)
- ▸ **Maximum Heart Rate:** 115 beats per minute (test stopped due to dyspnea)

- **Resting Heart Rate:** 85 bpm
- **Peak Blood Pressure:** 150/90 mm Hg
- **Resting Blood Pressure:** 100/80 mm Hg
- $\dot{V}O_2$**max**: 12 ml·min^{-1}·kg^{-1}

After meeting with Mr. E., you decide to prescribe a low-intensity exercise program using the FITT principle and following ACSM guidelines (Franklin 2000; Myers 1997).

Frequency: Many patients with chronic CHF such as Mr. E. become very tired after exercise. Exercise sessions of three to seven days per week are recommended.

Intensity: A target heart rate corresponding to 40-75% of $\dot{V}O_2$max or an RPE of 11-14 is standard. Note that the ACSM has changed the basis for cardiorespiratory exercise prescription from %$\dot{V}O_2$max to %$\dot{V}O_2$R for most situations; however, at this time, it has retained the terminology of %$\dot{V}O_2$max for certain special populations (Franklin 2000). Because Mr. E. performed very poorly on his modified Bruce treadmill test, and dyspnea was the limiting factor, you prescribe exercise based on an RPE of 11-14 rather than determining a target HR. Mr. E. will need to tailor his intensity according to his dyspnea (for more information on dyspnea, see case study 10.2).

Time: After a prolonged warm-up period of 10-15 minutes, exercise intervals as brief as 2-6 minutes may be required. Initially you set a goal of 10-20 minutes for Mr. E., with instructions to progressively lengthen this period to 40 minutes.

Type: You prescribe walking, stationary cycling, and other aerobic activities that can be well tolerated. Later, Mr. E. can add resistance training using high repetitions and low weight, no more frequently than three days per week.

PACEMAKERS

Exercise recommendations vary according to the type of pacemaker. The first type of pacemaker—represented by the acronym VVI—is used to manage **ventricular bradycardias.** The disadvantage of this device is that it does not allow the heart rate, and therefore cardiac output, to increase normally during exercise. The pacemaker is set at a fixed heart rate, so exercise prescriptions using target heart rates are inappropriate. For a complete description of pacemakers and their codes, see the reference by Franklin (2000).

The second type of pacemaker is **rate-responsive** and rate-modulated, allowing heart rate and cardiac output to increase with exercise. This type of pacemaker—the acronym is DDDR or VVIR—most closely mimics the heart's normal control. For these patients, exercise can be prescribed using a target heart rate, as well as by workload based on a $\dot{V}O_2$ or RPE.

The final type of pacemaker is an **antitachycardic** pacemaker, or ICD. These pacemakers manage rapid heart rates by delivering an electric shock to the heart. You can use standard ACSM guidelines to prescribe exercise for these patients—just be certain that you know the upper limits of the ICD, so you won't prescribe a heart rate that will elicit inappropriate shocks during exercise!

CASE STUDY 8.3
Patient With Pacemaker

Cecelia P. has recently had a VVI pacemaker installed to manage ventricular bradycardia. Ms. P. had been feeling very tired, which brought this condition to the attention of a physician. As a result of the nature of Ms. P.'s pacemaker, her heart rate is set at a fixed rate of 120 beats per minute. Her resting and peak blood pressures are 100/80 and 140/84 mmHg, respectively. She has been referred to your phase III/IV outpatient cardiac rehabilitation program for exercise.

Following ACSM guidelines, you develop the following exercise prescription for Ms. P. with the FITT principle (Franklin 2000).

Frequency: You recommend four to seven days per week and encourage her to be active on days outside of her rehabilitation session.

Intensity: An intensity of 50-85% of HRR can be used for patients with rate-responsive pacemakers. But Ms. P. has a fixed-rate pacemaker and will not demonstrate a linear relationship between heart rate and oxygen consumption. Prescribing exercise by target heart rate is not appropriate. You can prescribe intensity according to RPE, a target workload based on $\dot{V}O_2$, or a modified Karvonen formula for blood pressure. The modified Karvonen formula substitutes **systolic blood pressure (SBP)** in place of heart rate. The following is a calculation of target systolic blood pressure for Ms. P. at 50% and 85% intensities, using a modified Karvonen formula:

Target SBP = (intensity fraction)(SBPmax − SBPrest) + SBPrest

Lower target SBP = (0.50)(140 − 100) + 100

= (0.50)(40) + 100

= 20 + 100

= 120 mmHg

Upper target SBP = (0.85)(140 − 100) + 100

= (0.85)(40) + 100

= 34 + 100

= 134 mmHg

Time: Most phase III/IV cardiac rehabilitation programs consist of 60-minute time slots for exercise. You prescribe interval training at first, followed by progressive increases in exercise time to achieve 20-60 minutes per session.

Type: You prescribe walking, cycling, swimming, and other aerobic activities that involve large muscle groups. Low- to moderate-intensity resistance training may be indicated but should not begin until two to three weeks after implantation of the pacemaker to avoid dislodging implanted leads.

CARDIAC TRANSPLANT

Individuals with severe, untreatable cardiac disease, such as advanced congestive heart failure, may be eligible for cardiac transplantation. Donor hearts are in very short supply. Transplant recipients present a unique situation to the exercise professional. Of special concern are the physiological responses of the denervated heart, as well as the possibility of tissue rejection.

CASE STUDY 8.4
Cardiac Transplant Patient

Phillip E., the 65-year-old retired salesman described in case study 8.2 with a history of congestive heart failure, became a candidate for a cardiac transplant because his condition had progressed to end-stage heart failure. After his transplant, Mr. E. was referred to your phase II cardiac rehabilitation program for exercise.

(continued)

Case Study 8.4   *(continued)*

Using the FITT principle, and following ACSM guidelines, you devise the following exercise prescription:

Frequency: Mr. E. should do aerobic exercise four to six days per week. (Encourage people enrolled in rehabilitation programs that meet only three days per week to exercise on off days. They can perform range-of-motion and resistance training two to three days per week.)

Intensity: Because transplantation surgery denervates the heart, heart rate does not increase during exercise (other than a small increase over time due to circulating catecholamines). You therefore cannot prescribe exercise by heart rate. The ACSM recommends that you set exercise intensity at a target workload based on 50-75% peak $\dot{V}O_2$ or an RPE of 11-15 (Franklin 2000; Ketayian and Brawner 1997). If cardiopulmonary data are available, you can base the intensity on the ventilatory threshold. In some cases, you may need to use the dyspnea scale (table 10.2). Mr. E. was unable to perform a maximal cardiorespiratory exercise test because of early exhaustion, so you can base his exercise intensity on the RPE scale using a range of 11-15.

Time: You indicate that Mr. E. should begin his sessions with at least 15 minutes of continuous exercise, progressing to 60 minutes.

Type: Any aerobic exercise that works large muscle groups is appropriate—e.g., walking, jogging, cycling, swimming, stepping, and rowing. You also encourage Mr. E. to engage in resistance training to prevent glucocorticoid-induced myopathy and loss of lean body mass.

During exercise, supervision should focus on recognizing the adverse effects of immunosuppressive drug therapy and on recognizing the possibility of rejection. *Some important possible consequences of immunosuppressive therapy include hypertension, loss of muscle mass, glucose intolerance, and osteoporosis.* If any sign of rejection is noted, Mr. E. should discontinue his exercise until the rejection is reversed.

REFERENCES

1. Franklin, BA, ed. 2000. *ACSM's Guidelines for Exercise Testing and Prescription*, 6th ed., 165-199. Philadelphia: Lippincott Williams & Wilkins.

2. Ketayian, SJ, and C Brawner. 1997. Cardiac transplant. In *ACSM's Exercise Management for Persons With Chronic Diseases and Disabilities*, ed. JL Durstine, 54-58. Champaign, IL: Human Kinetics.

3. Myers, JN. 1997. Congestive heart failure. In *ACSM's Exercise Management for Persons With Chronic Diseases and Disabilities*, ed. JL Durstine, 48-53. Champaign, IL: Human Kinetics.

4. Ornish, D, SE Brown, LW Scherwitz, JH Billings, WT Armstrong, TA Ports, and SM McLanahan. 1990. Can lifestyle changes reverse coronary heart disease? The Lifestyle Heart Trial. *Lancet* 336:129-133.

5. Pollock, ML, GA Gaesser, JD Butcher, JP Despres, RK Dishman, BA Franklin, and CE Garber. 1998. The recommended quantity and quality of exercise for developing and maintaining cardiorespiratory and muscular fitness, and flexibility in healthy adults (ACSM position stand). *Med. Sci. Sports Exerc.* 30:975-991.

6. Wenger, KN, and HK Hellerstein. 1992. *Rehabilitation of the Coronary Patient*, 3rd ed., 25-26. New York: Churchill Livingston.

CHAPTER

9

Exercise Prescription for Diabetes Mellitus

Exercise is highly valuable in the treatment of diabetes, but its impact is affected by the type of diabetes that the client has. There are two principal types of diabetes mellitus. Type 1 is a relatively rare disorder that usually begins in childhood, when the individual's immune system destroys the insulin-producing cells of the pancreas. As a result, glucose cannot enter most cells in the body and builds up in the bloodstream. The individual must inject insulin regularly for survival. Type 1 diabetes was formerly known as juvenile-onset, or as insulin-dependent diabetes mellitus (IDDM).

Type 2 diabetes is much more common, accounting for over 90% of all cases of diabetes. In type 2 diabetes, cells throughout the body become less sensitive to insulin. Insulin is still made by the pancreas, but it is progressively less effective at moving glucose into the cells. This loss of insulin sensitivity is strongly related to both inactivity and obesity. Type 2 diabetes was once found almost exclusively in middle-aged or older adults, but with the growing obesity epidemic it is becoming increasingly more common in children. Type 2 diabetes was formerly known as adult-onset, or as noninsulin-dependent diabetes mellitus (NIDDM). The latter term was especially misleading because many type 2 patients "progress" in their treatment from (1) exercise and diet, to (2) oral drugs that stimulate insulin secretion, to (3) insulin injections. Thus, some type 2 patients are in fact "dependent" on exogenous insulin.

Other categories of diabetes mellitus that are closely related to type 2 are impaired fasting glucose (IFG), impaired glucose tolerance (IGT), and gestational diabetes mellitus (GDM). IFG and IGT are related terms that signify the early stage of type 2 diabetes, before a person reaches the criteria for a diagnosis of diabetes. Diabetes is usually diagnosed as fasting blood glucose levels ≥ 126 mg·dl^{-1}, but it can also be diagnosed from symptoms and random blood glucose values or from the results of a glucose tolerance test (Expert Committee 1997). **Impaired fasting glucose** is defined as fasting blood glucose levels from 110-125 mg·dl^{-1}. **Impaired glucose tolerance** is basically the same condition as IFG, but is based on the results of a glucose tolerance test rather than fasting blood glucose. For a glucose tolerance test, the individual drinks a glucose solution and blood glucose is measured over the next three hours to observe how high it rises. Criteria are then used to diagnosis diabetes or the less severe IGT (Expert Committee 1997). **Gestational diabetes mellitus** occurs in a small percentage of women during pregnancy. It usually ends after the pregnancy, but women who experience GDM have a higher risk of developing diabetes later in life.

Exercise therapy for clients with type 1 diabetes is aimed primarily at reducing the risk of cardiovascular disease and improving overall fitness. Exercise therapy for clients with type 2 diabetes is potentially a very effective treatment for the disease itself. Because exercise training improves insulin sensitivity (Devlin 1992), individuals with type 2 diabetes who exercise sufficiently often can normalize their blood glucose control. In one research study, five individuals with type 2 diabetes and 8 individuals with IGT entered a one-year exercise program (Holloszy et al. 1986). Over the year, they built up their exercise time to 50-60 minutes, five times per week, at 70-90% of maximal $\dot{V}O_2$. At the end of the year, three of the five patients with diabetes and all eight of the IGT patients had completely normalized their responses to glucose tolerance tests. Although exercise is highly effective at improving insulin sensitivity, like any fitness adaptation, the improved sensitivity regresses if regular exercise is not maintained (Albright et al. 2000).

EXERCISE PRESCRIPTION FOR CLIENTS WITH TYPE 1 DIABETES

You can use the standard ACSM exercise prescription guidelines for clients with diabetes (table 2.1). But people with diabetes are in the ACSM's high-risk category, and should be evaluated by a physician before starting an exercise program. Table 9.1 lists common secondary complications of diabetes that should be considered in the medical evaluation (American Diabetes Association 2000; Franklin 2000).

Table 9.1

Medical Evaluation of Clients With Diabetes Prior to Exercise

Metabolic Control

The individual must have an acceptable level of glucose control (< 300 mg·dl^{-1}, preferably < 240 mg·dl^{-1}), through medication if needed, since exercise can worsen hyperglycemia.

Coronary Artery Disease

A stress test is needed in people >35 years old, or in those with additional risk factors, given the increased risk caused by diabetes. Beta-blockers may mask symptoms of hypoglycemia.

Retinopathy

If proliferative retinopathy or moderate to severe nonproliferative retinopathy is present, the individual must avoid exercises that jar the body or that induce a hypertensive response. Individuals who have undergone laser treatment must obtain approval of an ophthalmologist before proceeding with an exercise program.

Autonomic Neuropathy

Assess for orthostatic intolerance and use seated exercise if needed. The HR response to exercise is blunted. Avoid exercise in excessive heat.

Peripheral Neuropathy

Clean and examine feet regularly. Consider nonweightbearing exercise.

Nephropathy

Exercise capacity may be reduced. Thus, exercise intensity should be low.

Once people with diabetes enter an exercise program, help them take special care to avoid hypoglycemia—a risk particularly for individuals with type 1 diabetes. Because both insulin and exercise reduce blood glucose, there is the potential for a dangerous fall in blood glucose during and after exercise. Clients with type 1 diabetes who have a planned exercise routine should reduce the insulin dosage of the pre-exercise injection. Although individuals differ widely in their responses, a good starting point is to reduce the short-acting insulin taken prior to exercise by 30-50% (Colberg 2000; Colberg and Swain 2000). You can also suggest that your client increase carbohydrate intake prior to exercise; but note that the ACSM recommends decreasing insulin as the principal tool (Franklin 2000).

It is preferable to plan ahead, but people inevitably decide on impulse to go out for a run or a game of tennis. People with type 1 diabetes who are about to engage in unplanned exercise should consider consuming 20-30 g of carbohydrates for each 30 minutes of anticipated exercise in order to prevent a fall in blood glucose during the exercise. Everyone with diabetes, regardless of the type, should have a fast-acting source of sugar (juice, hard candy, etc.) available during exercise to consume immediately if hypoglycemic symptoms occur (weakness, lightheadedness, etc.). Hypoglycemia requires immediate attention, as it can quickly become life-threatening. One or two pieces of hard candy or a small glass of juice should relieve symptoms in less than five minutes. If someone loses consciousness, call 911 or whatever the emergency number is in your area. Prior to the arrival of emergency personnel, try squirting a sugar-containing gel (or even cake frosting) onto the inner surface of the unconscious person's cheek. Table 9.2 summarizes steps that should be taken to avoid hypoglycemia (American Diabetes Association 2000; Colberg 2000; Franklin 2000).

Exercise can exacerbate hyperglycemia and ketosis. To minimize the risk of either hyper- or hypoglycemia, patients should monitor their blood glucose frequently at the start of a new exercise program. They should check blood glucose immediately before exercise and evaluate it using the information in table 9.3 (American Diabetes Association 2000; Franklin 2000). And they should also check it after exercise: if it is rising, they should consult their physician (unless it is rising due to consuming carbohydrates dur-

Table 9.2

Steps to Avoid Hypoglycemia*

Prior to Planned Exercise

Reduce pre-exercise insulin—amount based on individual responsiveness.

Prior to Unplanned Exercise

Consume 20-30 g carbohydrates (insulin users only).

Prior to Any Exercise

Consume 20-30 g carbohydrates if blood glucose < 100 mg·dl^{-1}.

During Exercise

Consume 20-30 g carbohydrates each 30 min for extended exercise (insulin users only).
Be aware of symptoms of hypoglycemia.
Exercise with a partner.
Carry fast-acting sugar and consume as needed if hypoglycemia occurs.

After Exercise

Consume 20-30 g carbohydrates if blood glucose < 100 mg·dl^{-1}.
Be aware of the potential for hypoglycemia for several hours.

* Note: These are guidelines only. They must be adapted to clients on an individual basis.

ing the exercise session). A rising blood glucose suggests that the patient may need an insulin injection, *to be determined by the physician,* in order to prevent ketosis and a possible diabetic coma. This is a much rarer consequence of exercise than is hypoglycemia, but both you and the patients with whom you work should be aware of the possibility. The postexercise value should be no more than the pre-exercise value. Some decrease is normal, but if it has fallen much more than is typical for a particular person, or has fallen below 100 mg·dl^{-1}, then he or she should consume extra carbohydrates.

With proper attention to the details of glucose and insulin management, people with type 1 diabetes can enjoy vigorous athletic pursuits (Colberg 2000).

Table 9.3	
Interpreting Blood Glucose Values Prior to Exercise	
If > 300 mg·dl⁻¹	Postpone exercise, consult physician/inject insulin.
If > 240 mg·dl⁻¹*	Check for urinary ketones; if present, postpone exercise, consult physician/inject insulin.
If 100-240 mg·dl⁻¹	OK to begin exercise.
If < 100 mg·dl⁻¹	Consume 20-30 g carbohydrates prior to exercising.

* 240 mg·dl⁻¹ is the value used by the ACSM in its 6th edition *Guidelines* (Franklin 2000). Other authorities use 250 mg·dl⁻¹ (American Diabetes Association 2000).

CASE STUDY 9.1
Client With Type 1 Diabetes Mellitus

Sheri C. is a 17-year-old high school distance runner. Over the past few weeks she began experiencing a number of unusual symptoms. The first symptom she noticed was that she had to get up during the night to urinate, eventually having to do this several times each night. She became thirsty all the time, even though she drank lots of water. She started losing weight and at the same time experienced an increase in her appetite. It seemed that no matter how much she ate, she still kept losing weight. Furthermore, her workouts were suffering. She felt constantly tired and lethargic, and her performance times were worsening even though she continued her regular training. Her family physician found her blood glucose to be 380 mg·dl⁻¹. The physician diagnosed her with type 1 diabetes mellitus and placed her on a twice-daily regimen of insulin injections, each injection consisting of both intermediate-acting (NPH) and short-acting (Humalog) insulin. Over the three months since her diagnosis, she has experienced several bouts of hypoglycemia, and her physician has modified her insulin dosage until her glucose levels have become fairly stable. During this time, she has been prohibited from running. She is now ready to resume her running, and her physician has referred her to you for advice and an exercise prescription. Her resting HR is 56 bpm, and her maximal HR measured during training is 194 bpm.

Ms. C. needs to return *gradually* to her former competitive training level, as would anyone coming back from a three-month layoff. You prescribe three exercise sessions per week at the beginning, on alternate days. Her previous training runs were over an hour long, but your initial prudent goal is 30 minutes. You set her intensity at a moderate level, which she is probably very capable of judging by her personal feelings of perceived exertion. However, to keep her from overdoing it at first, you provide a target HR range at 50-70% of HRR. Her maximal HR is 194 bpm, so use that value in the calculation of target HR, rather than 220 – age.

$$\text{Target HR} = (\text{intensity fraction})(\text{HRmax} - \text{HRrest}) + \text{HRrest}$$
$$\text{Lower target HR} = 0.50(194 - 56) + 56$$
$$= 0.50(138) + 56$$
$$= 69 + 56$$
$$= 125 \text{ bpm}$$
$$\text{Upper target HR} = 0.70(194 - 56) + 56$$
$$= 0.70(138) + 56$$
$$= 97 + 56$$
$$= 153 \text{ bpm}$$

Ms. C. should already be monitoring her blood glucose several times a day. If she is not, she needs to now. Ask her to measure her blood glucose when she wakes up. If the reading is her typical morning value, she should take her morning (prebreakfast) insulin injection, but she should reduce the dosage of short-acting insulin (Humalog) by 50% if she plans to exercise within one to two hours. If her exercise session will be in the afternoon, she should reduce the intermediate-acting insulin (NPH) instead, which does not reach peak levels in the bloodstream for at least four hours. After her usual breakfast, she should wait about an hour before starting preparations for her first run. Immediately before the run, she should measure her blood glucose again. During the run, she should carry a fast-acting sugar source and must pay attention to possible symptoms of hypoglycemia. Inform her that exercise can mask or change her usual hypoglycemic symptoms. Until her pattern is well established, she may need to arrange to check her blood glucose levels halfway through her run

(continued)

Case Study 9.1   *(continued)*

as well. After the run, she should measure her blood glucose again, and, if necessary, consume a carbohydrate snack at that time. If her postexercise blood glucose is less than 100 mg·dl⁻¹, or if she experiences any symptoms of hypoglycemia during or closely following her run, ask her to further reduce her pre-exercise insulin dosage for the exercise session two days from now. If her postexercise glucose is higher than her pre-exercise glucose, she will need to moderate the reduction in pre-exercise insulin. Instruct her to pay close attention to the possible development of hypoglycemia over the next couple of hours leading up to lunch time and even up to 24 hours after her running while she is unaccustomed to it. If she experiences nocturnal bouts of hypoglycemia following training days, then she will need to reduce her evening dose of intermediate-acting insulin (NPH) as well or consume an additional bedtime snack to compensate.

Ms. C. also needs to be aware of several other effects from regular training: (1) Her overall insulin needs may decrease with her regular activity, and she may need to reduce her intermediate-acting insulin (NPH) in addition to reducing her short-acting insulin (Humalog) during the training season if her food intake does not increase enough to compensate. (2) Training can increase her body's ability to use fat as fuel, and her blood sugars may begin to drop less during an activity once she has become accustomed to it. (3) Successive days of heavy exercise increase her risk for hypoglycemia, especially during the night. She may need to monitor her blood glucose levels during the night in this case, adjust her evening insulin doses, or eat an additional snack at bedtime. Using this approach, you can continue to help Ms. C. fine-tune her insulin regimen as she increases her training frequency, duration, and intensity back to her previous level. It is critical for her to recognize the importance of balancing a regular regimen of training with changes in insulin and diet to accomplish this successfully.

EXERCISE PRESCRIPTION FOR CLIENTS WITH TYPE 2 DIABETES

The principal goal for prescribing exercise for clients with type 2 diabetes is to burn calories. Most individuals with type 2 diabetes are obese, and burning calories attacks the diabetes twice: first, by improving tissue sensitivity to insulin; second, by reducing body fat. The exercise prescription therefore should focus on increasing the duration and frequency of exercise, using an intensity level that the client can sustain for long periods of time. For best results, gradually increase the duration and frequency to one hour, seven days per week. Two 30-minute sessions per day or three 20-minute sessions are perfectly acceptable ways to accomplish the same goal. Use these same guidelines to prescribe exercise for individuals with impaired fasting glucose or impaired glucose tolerance. Women with gestational diabetes also need an exercise prescription that focuses on calorie burning, but this must be tempered as needed with concerns associated with pregnancy itself (see chapter 10).

Because most clients with type 2 diabetes start out with a low fitness level, prescribe light to moderate exercise intensity—e.g., 40-60% of $\dot{V}O_2R$. A greater intensity will burn more calories, but it is less likely to be sustained long enough to burn as many calories as a more moderate intensity. Moreover, high-intensity programs may lead to a greater dropout rate than those requiring only moderate intensities. Despite the drawbacks of high-intensity prescriptions, however, it is still a good idea to encourage clients to increase the intensity *within their level of tolerance* as their programs progress.

Clients with type 2 diabetes are much less likely than those with type 1 diabetes to experience either hypoglycemia or hyperglycemia as a result of exercise. The exception is type 2 clients who take insulin: their responses are much more like those with type 1 diabetes, and you should handle them accordingly. Hypoglycemia is comparatively rare with type 2 diabetes, but be sure that all such clients are aware of its potential, remain alert to its symptoms, and carry a fast-acting source of sugar during exercise.

Individuals with type 2 diabetes are just as susceptible as those with type 1 to the secondary complications listed in table 9.1. It is imperative that they be evaluated by a physician prior to starting an exercise program.

CASE STUDY 9.2
Client With Type 2 Diabetes Mellitus

Rudy B. is 72 years old, 5'10" tall, and weighs 278 lb. He was diagnosed with type 2 diabetes five years ago and has been treated

(continued)

Case Study 9.2   *(continued)*

with oral hypoglycemic agents. His physician has told him that he must do a better job with diet and exercise or eventually he will have to go on insulin. He gets no regular exercise and his diet consists largely of red meats, fried foods, and creamy sauces. At his last medical checkup, Mr. B. had a total cholesterol of 264 mg·dl⁻¹, LDL 145 mg·dl⁻¹, HDL 38 mg·dl⁻¹, and fasting glucose was 156 mg·dl⁻¹. Because of his high risk of heart disease, he was given a stress test. He completed a cycling protocol up to 140 W, obtaining a maximal HR of 160 bpm. His resting HR is 78 bpm. There were no signs of coronary ischemia. His physician reports that he has no other overt medical conditions at this time and has referred him to your facility for lifestyle modification and an exercise prescription. Mr. B. rarely monitors his blood sugar. He says it is too expensive for him to buy strips.

Mr. B. is quite typical of individuals with type 2 diabetes. He is obese (BMI of 40 kg·m⁻²), has elevated LDL (and total) cholesterol, is sedentary, and has only moderate control over his blood glucose levels. These factors all greatly raise his risk of heart disease. Fortunately, he does not yet exhibit clinically significant heart disease. Encourage him to set a goal of reaching a target weight at a BMI of 25 kg·m⁻², which would be about 174 lb. Losing approximately 100 pounds of fat will take one year of consistent exercise and dietary discipline. He should reduce his caloric intake by about 500 kcal per day, primarily through selecting foods that are lower in fat than he currently chooses.

You begin his exercise prescription with 20-minute sessions, three times per week, at 40-60% of $\dot{V}O_2R$. You can use a target HR range or a target workload to establish the intensity. Over the next few weeks, he needs to increase the frequency and duration of his exercise to an effective level—i.e., to one hour daily if he is willing. Your primary task is to convince Mr. B. of the value of performing this much exercise. His target HR would be as follows:

$$\text{Target HR} = (\text{intensity fraction})(\text{HRmax} - \text{HRrest}) + \text{HRrest}$$
$$\text{Lower target HR} = (0.40)(160 - 78) + 78$$
$$= (0.40)(82) + 78$$
$$= 33 + 78$$
$$= 111 \text{ bpm}$$

$$\text{Upper target HR} = (0.60)(160 - 78) + 78$$
$$= (0.60)(82) + 78$$
$$= 49 + 78$$
$$= 127 \text{ bpm}$$

You could determine his target workload by (1) estimating his $\dot{V}O_2$max from his maximal workload of 140 W, (2) determining the target $\dot{V}O_2$ at 40-60% of $\dot{V}O_2$R, and then (3) converting the target $\dot{V}O_2$ into the target workload. It is simpler just to take 40-60% of the maximal workload itself:

$$\text{Lower target workload} = (0.40)(140 \text{ W})$$
$$= 56 \text{ W}$$
$$\text{Upper target workload} = (0.60)(140 \text{ W})$$
$$= 84 \text{ W}$$

Thus, you gauge his exercise intensity as a HR between 111 and 127 bpm or as a workload between 56 and 84 W. To determine a workload on a piece of equipment that does not indicate the power in watts, such as a treadmill, you would need to go through the three steps described above for converting to a $\dot{V}O_2$ and then back to a workload.

How many net calories will Mr. B. burn with his exercise program? Using the 84 W ($84 \times 6 = 504$ kg·m·min^{-1}) workload at his current body weight of 287 lb ($287/2.2 = 130.5$ kg), you obtain the following:

$$\dot{V}O_2 = 7 + 1.8(\text{workload})/(\text{body mass})$$
$$= 7 + 1.8(504)/130.5$$
$$= 7 + 907.2/130.5$$
$$= 7 + 7.0$$
$$= 14 \text{ ml·min}^{-1}\text{·kg}^{-1}$$
$$\text{net } \dot{V}O_2 = 14 - 3.5 = 10.5 \text{ ml·min}^{-1}\text{·kg}^{-1}$$
$$(10.5 \text{ ml·min}^{-1}\text{·kg}^{-1})(130.5 \text{ kg})/1000 = 1.37 \text{ L·min}^{-1}$$
$$(1.37 \text{ L·min}^{-1}) \times (5 \text{ kcal·L}^{-1}) = 6.85 \text{ kcal·min}^{-1}$$

If he burns a net 6.85 kcal per minute for 30 minutes, three times a week, this would total $6.85 \times 30 \times 3 = 617$ kcal per week. There

(continued)

Case Study 9.2 *(continued)*

are 3,500 kcal stored in a pound of fat, so he would be losing 617/3500 = 0.18 lb, or less than one fifth of a pound per week through the exercise. However, if he does his exercises for 60 minutes, 7 times per week, it would total 6.85 × 60 × 7 = 2,877 kcal per week. This is a little more than four fifths of a pound of fat each week (2877/3500 = 0.82 lb). He has also been asked to reduce his caloric intake by 500 kcal per day (i.e., 3,500 kcal, or 1 lb per week), so he should be losing nearly 2 pounds per week with this program. Be sure to reevaluate his status every three months and modify his program as appropriate. Although at some point in the future you should consider incorporating resistance training into his program, for the time being Mr. B. needs to focus his available time on burning calories.

Mr. B. is reluctant to monitor his blood glucose, in part because of the financial cost. It is imperative, however, that he monitor his blood glucose before and after each exercise session when he first begins the program. Once he establishes a steady response pattern, it would be acceptable for him to reduce his monitoring to one exercise session per week. However, as with all patients with diabetes, *it would be better if he would monitor several times daily*. As his condition improves, his current level of hypoglycemic medication may be too much. He will need to be aware of the growing possibility of hypoglycemia, and his physician will probably have to reduce his medication as the year progresses. It is quite possible that he will be able to get off his medication entirely.

CASE STUDY 9.3

Type 2 Client With Secondary Complications

Juanita L. is 56 years old, 5'1" tall, and weighs 192 lb. She was diagnosed with type 2 diabetes at age 38 and has injected insulin twice daily for the past seven years. She has had ulcers on her feet that are currently healed, and she has been diagnosed with peripheral neuropathy. She has moderate nonproliferative retinopathy. She was given an arm ergometry stress test recently, and her $\dot{V}O_2$max was measured at 11 ml·min^{-1}·kg^{-1}, with a maximal HR of 152 bpm. Her resting HR is 92 bpm. She exhibited 2 mm of ST depression at maximal exercise but no abnormal heart rhythms or symptoms of ischemia. On follow-up, an angiogram revealed mild blockage of two coronary arteries—for which she currently takes aspirin and beta-blockers. She has been referred to your facility for exercise training.

In creating an exercise prescription for Ms. L., you need to consider the secondary complications of her diabetes. *Peripheral neuropathy:* She has poor sensation in her feet, and she will need to inspect and clean her feet at least once a day and immediately after each exercise session. She may need to select exercises that require her feet to bear less weight, based on her level of tolerance. Walking is a possibility, but she may have to use stationary cycling or rowing or possibly even arm ergometry. *Retinopathy:* She must avoid exercises that entail jarring or large increases in blood pressure. Jarring should not be a problem because you are already limiting her weightbearing exercises because of her foot problems. To avoid excessive increases in blood pressure, instruct her to avoid the Valsalva maneuver during resistance training and to consider using a lighter weight that she can lift 10-15 times without going to failure. *Coronary heart disease:* Because she performed her stress test before she was placed on beta-blockers, you can't use the HR data that were collected at that time to establish target HRs. If she does another stress test while on her medication, you can use that information to determine target HRs, as the HR response to exercise under beta-blockade is still linear. For the time being, use RPE or target workload to establish intensity. Begin her exercise prescription at 40-60% of $\dot{V}O_2R$ for 20-30 minutes, three times per week. Table 3.1 shows that an intensity of 40-60% of $\dot{V}O_2R$ corresponds to an RPE of 12-14. Target workloads using arm ergometry are calculated here.

$$\text{Target } \dot{V}O_2 = (\text{intensity fraction})(\dot{V}O_2\text{max} - 3.5) + 3.5$$
$$\text{Lower target } \dot{V}O_2 = (0.40)(11 - 3.5) + 3.5$$
$$= (0.40)(7.5) + 3.5$$
$$= 3.0 + 3.5$$
$$= 6.5 \text{ ml·min}^{-1}\text{·kg}^{-1}$$
$$\text{Upper target } \dot{V}O_2 = (0.60)(11 - 3.5) + 3.5$$
$$= (0.60)(7.5) + 3.5$$
$$= 4.5 + 3.5$$
$$= 8.0 \text{ ml·min}^{-1}\text{·kg}^{-1}$$

(continued)

Case Study 9.3   *(continued)*

Now, determine the corresponding workloads on an arm ergometer.

$$\dot{V}O_2 = 3.5 + 3(\text{work rate})/(\text{body mass})$$

Lower target workload:

$$6.5 = 3.5 + 3(\text{work rate})/87.3$$
$$6.5 - 3.5 = 3(\text{work rate})/87.3$$
$$3.0 = 3(\text{work rate})/87.3$$
$$3/3 = (\text{work rate})/87.3$$
$$1.0 = (\text{work rate})/87.3$$
$$87.3 \text{ kg·m·min}^{-1} = \text{work rate}$$

Upper target workload:

$$8.0 = 3.5 + 3(\text{work rate})/87.3$$
$$8.0 - 3.5 = 3(\text{work rate})/87.3$$
$$4.5 = 3(\text{work rate})/87.3$$
$$4.5/3 = (\text{work rate})/87.3$$
$$1.5 = (\text{work rate})/87.3$$
$$1.5 \times 87.3 = \text{work rate}$$
$$131 \text{ kg·m·min}^{-1} = \text{work rate}$$

What would be the resistance setting if she uses a Monark arm ergometer (2.4 m flywheel distance) at a cadence of 50 rpm? Use the cycle ergometer work rate equation from chapter 4, page 57.

Work rate = (resistance setting)(flywheel distance per rev)(rpm)

Lower target workload:

$$87 = (\text{resistance setting})(2.4)(50)$$
$$87 = (\text{resistance setting})(120)$$
$$87/120 = \text{resistance setting}$$
$$0.73 \text{ kg} = \text{resistance setting}$$

Upper target workload:

$$131 = (\text{resistance setting})(120)$$
$$131/120 = \text{resistance setting}$$
$$1.09 \text{ kg} = \text{resistance setting}$$

Ms. L. should use a resistance setting of about 0.7 to 1.1 kg on the arm ergometer if she is cranking at 50 rpm.

Ms. L. is obese (BMI of 36 $kg \cdot m^{-2}$) and would benefit from a structured weight loss program. Because she uses insulin, you will need to increase the frequency and duration of her exercise very carefully. As with the type 1 diabetic in case study 9.1, Ms. L. will need to reduce her pre-exercise insulin dosage and pay special attention to the risk of hypoglycemia during exercise.

REFERENCES

1. Albright, A, M Franz, G Hornsby, A Kriska, D Marrero, I Ullrich, and LS Verity. 2000. Exercise and type 2 diabetes (ACSM Position Stand). *Med. Sci. Sports Exerc.* 32:1345-1360.

2. American Diabetes Association. 2000. Diabetes mellitus and exercise—position statement. *Diab. Care* 23(Suppl 1):S50-54.

3. Colberg, SR. 2000. *The Diabetic Athlete.* Champaign, IL: Human Kinetics.

4. Colberg, SR, and DP Swain. 2000. Exercise and diabetes control. *Physician Sportsmed.* 28(4):63-81.

5. Devlin, JT. 1992. Effects of exercise on insulin sensitivity in humans. *Diab. Care* 15:1690-1693.

6. Expert Committee. 1997. Report of the Expert Committee on the diagnosis and classification of diabetes mellitus. *Diab. Care* 20:1183-1197.

7. Franklin, BA, ed. 2000. *ACSM's Guidelines for Exercise Testing and Prescription,* 6th ed., 211-214. Philadelphia: Lippincott Williams & Wilkins.

8. Holloszy, JO, J Schultz, J Kusnierkiewicz, JM Hagberg, and AA Ehsani. 1986. Effect of exercise on glucose tolerance and insulin resistance. *Acta Med. Scand.* 711(Suppl):55-65.

CHAPTER
10

Exercise Prescription for Other Special Cases

This chapter discusses ACSM exercise prescriptions for a variety of special cases, some of which are clinical conditions that are routinely associated together in the same patient: peripheral vascular disease (PVD), chronic obstructive pulmonary disease (COPD), and hypertension (HTN). In addition, it covers the special cases of exercise during pregnancy and exercise prescription for children.

PERIPHERAL VASCULAR DISEASE

Peripheral vascular disease (PVD), sometimes referred to as peripheral arterial disease (PAD), is a condition that results in occlusion or blockage of the arteries of the lower extremities. This results in insufficient blood flow, lactic acid accumulation, and a burning pain in the affected muscles, such as the calves. Ten percent of adults over 70 years of age have signs/symptoms of PVD.

CASE STUDY 10.1
Client With Peripheral Vascular Disease

Juan S. is a 60-year-old male who suffers from peripheral vascular disease (PVD) and moderate chronic obstructive pulmonary disease (COPD). He has been unsuccessful in smoking cessation programs and currently smokes between one and two packs of cigarettes per day. Many individuals with PVD smoke, and Mr. S.'s history of smoking has probably resulted in his COPD. During a treadmill test, Mr. S. could walk at only 2 mph for 30 seconds when he developed severe, burning leg pain in the calf that forced him to stop. Doppler studies revealed ankle-to-arm pressure indexes less than 0.90 at rest (i.e., ankle systolic BP is less than 90% of brachial systolic BP). He was then given an arm ergometer test. Results of this test were as follows:

- **ECG:** Normal sinus rhythm
- **Peak heart rate:** 130 bpm
- **Resting heart rate:** 75 bpm
- **Peak blood pressure:** 148/92 mmHg
- **Resting blood pressure:** 128/86 mmHg
- **S_aO_2 at peak exercise:** 93%
- **Peak work rate:** 60 W

Whenever an individual presents with more than one chronic condition, you should focus the exercise prescription on the most severe condition. Mr. S.'s PVD is quite serious, based on his pain during walking and his poor ankle-to-arm systolic index. His COPD is less serious, because his arterial oxygen saturation (S_aO_2) does not drop below 88% during exercise. Therefore, because his ability to exercise is limited by his PVD and not his COPD, focus Mr. S.'s exercise prescription on his PVD using the FITT principle and following ACSM recommendations (Franklin 2000; Gardner 1997).

Frequency: The frequency of exercise should be at least three days per week. However, for individuals where exercise may be intermittent and of low intensity, daily exercise is recommended to maximize improvements.

Intensity: An intensity of 40-70% of $\dot{V}O_2$max is recommended. Note that the ACSM has changed the basis for cardiorespiratory exercise prescription from %$\dot{V}O_2$max to %$\dot{V}O_2$R for most situations; however, it has still retained the terminology of % $\dot{V}O_2$max for certain special populations (Franklin 2000). In Mr. S.'s case, exercise prescription based on $\dot{V}O_2$ would be appropriate only for arm exercise, because his HR and $\dot{V}O_2$ responses to leg exercise are not known. The peak HR and $\dot{V}O_2$ during arm exercise are generally much less than during leg exercise. For performing leg exercise, Mr. S. should exercise until he reaches a pain level of 3 out of 4 on the claudication scale (table 10.1) and then rest until he is able to resume exercise. In this way, he will be able to increase his exercise tolerance.

Time: You prescribe 20-40 minutes of continuous exercise per

Table 10.1	
Claudication Scale	
Grade 1	Minimal pain or discomfort
Grade 2	Moderate pain or discomfort, but attention can be diverted
Grade 3	Intense pain, attention cannot be diverted
Grade 4	Excruciating pain, cannot continue

Adapted, by permission, from *ACSM's Guidelines For Exercise Testing and Prescription*, 6th ed., 2000, edited by BA Franklin (Philadelphia: Lippincott Williams & Wilkins), 209.

session. You tell Mr. S. that he need not achieve this amount in one continuous exercise bout, but he may perform multiple discontinuous bouts as his comfort level permits.

Type: You recommend weightbearing exercise such as walking to improve circulation in Mr. S.'s lower limbs. However, you point out that he can extend his exercise session by replacing rest periods with nonweightbearing activities such as cycling, swimming, or arm ergometry—that way he can maintain the intensity and increase the duration of his exercise, thereby improving his cardiovascular fitness.

To conclude the case study, assume that Mr. S. has progressed and is now able to do 20 minutes of continuous exercise and can complete a treadmill exercise test. This is an important milestone, because his earlier arm ergometry test may not have reached a

(continued)

Case Study 10.1   *(continued)*

high enough intensity to reveal underlying heart disease. You are now able to measure his cardiorespiratory fitness and can prescribe exercise using a target heart rate. His maximum heart rate is 150 beats per minute, achieved by walking 2 mph at a 10% grade. Metabolic data are not available. Calculate a target heart rate range for Mr. S. using the heart rate reserve method. First, calculate his $\dot{V}O_2$max using the walking equation from table 4.1, to be able to determine the appropriate intensity level to apply to his target heart rate range. His walking speed is (2 mph) $\times$ (26.8) = 53.6 m·min^{-1}.

$$\dot{V}O_2 = 3.5 + 0.1(\text{speed}) + 1.8(\text{speed})(\text{fractional grade})$$
$$= 3.5 + 0.1(53.6) + 1.8(53.6)(0.10)$$
$$= 3.5 + 5.36 + 9.648$$
$$= 18.5 \text{ ml·min}^{-1}\text{·kg}^{-1}$$

Mr. S.'s aerobic capacity is low—using the formula in table 4.2 ($\dot{V}O_2$ in ml·min·kg^{-1})/3.5 = $\dot{V}O_2$ in METs), we see that it is only (18.5 ml·min^{-1}·kg^{-1})/3.5 = 5.3 METs. You therefore use a heart rate range of 40-60%. Mr. S.'s resting heart rate is 75 beats per minute.

$$\text{Target HR} = (\text{intensity fraction})(\text{HRmax} - \text{HRrest}) + \text{HRrest}$$
$$\text{Lower target HR} = (0.40)(150 - 75) + 75$$
$$= (0.40)(75) + 75$$
$$= 30 + 75$$
$$= 105 \text{ bpm}$$
$$\text{Upper target HR} = (0.60)(150 - 75) + 75$$
$$= (0.60)(75) + 75$$
$$= 45 + 75$$
$$= 120 \text{ bpm}$$

CHRONIC OBSTRUCTIVE PULMONARY DISEASE

Chronic obstructive pulmonary disease is common in cigarette smokers and consists of emphysema, chronic bronchitis, or a combination of the two. Exercise benefits for individuals with COPD include increased exercise capacity, functional status, and quality of life, as well as a decrease in the severity of dyspnea. Individuals who have COPD or other lung diseases generally experience a gradual downhill prognosis. Rather than attempting to reverse the disease, exercise-based rehabilitation should aim to reduce the functional impairment.

CASE STUDY 10.2
Client With Chronic Obstructive Pulmonary Disease

Penelope C. is 60 years old, with a life-long history of cigarette smoking. She has severe chronic obstructive pulmonary disease (COPD), and her S_aO_2 falls below 88% when she exercises. She has been admitted to your pulmonary rehabilitation program for exercise conditioning.

Using the FITT principle and ACSM recommendations (Franklin 2000), you devise Ms. C's exercise prescription as follows:

Frequency: Most COPD exercise programs are hospital-based and range from one to five days per week, averaging two days, usually Tuesdays and Thursdays. Patients who are "end-stage" may be inconsistent in their ability to exercise. Therefore, you must consider patient variability and functional status when determining the frequency.

Intensity: Ms. C. desaturates during exercise, so it is important to use a pulse oximeter to monitor her arterial oxygen S_aO_2 to prevent it from falling below 88%. Should her S_aO_2 regularly fall below 88% when she is exercising at her prescribed intensity, you need to decrease the intensity and contact her physician. You may want to request that her physician prescribe a nasal oxygen cannula for Ms. C. to use during exercise. If metabolic data are available for Ms. C., you may want to prescribe her exercise at 50% of peak oxygen consumption. More likely, you will need to prescribe her intensity based on her symptoms. As with the PVD patient, she should exercise up to her level of tolerance and try to increase the duration of her intermittent bouts. One means of gauging her intensity would be by the use of a dyspnea scale, of which there are several in use. As an example, she could attempt to work at level 3 on the scale in table 10.2.

Time: Continuous exercise of 20 minutes or more would be desirable. However, as with PVD, accumulating this much time through repeated bouts of intermittent exercise is more

(continued)

Case Study 10.2 *(continued)*

Table 10.2

Dyspnea Scale

+1	Mild, noticeable to patient but not observer
+2	Mild, some difficulty noticeable to observer
+3	Moderate difficulty, can continue
+4	Severe difficulty, cannot continue

Adapted, by permission, from *ACSM's Guidelines For Exercise Testing and Prescription*, 4th ed., 1991, edited by RR Pate (Philadelphia: Lea & Febiger), 73.

appropriate for most patients, until they are able to tolerate continuous exercise.

Type: You should prescribe aerobic activities that involve large muscle groups, such as walking, cycling, and swimming. Aerobic exercise that focuses on smaller muscle groups, such as arm ergometry, may result in a higher ventilation and may be less well tolerated. You also will want to add strength training two to three days per week, especially for the upper body, using low resistance and high repetitions.

Instruct Ms. C. in pursed-lips breathing—i.e., she should inhale through her nose and exhale through a small gap between her lips. Because exhaling in this manner extends the time of the exhalation and requires more force, it potentially can keep airways more open. Ms. C. should use pursed-lips breathing not only during exercise but whenever she experiences dyspnea.

HYPERTENSION

Hypertension (HTN) is a major health problem in the United States and other Western industrialized countries. It has been estimated that there are as many as 50 million Americans with high blood pressure, many of whom are taking medications. **Hypertension** is defined as systolic blood pressure consistently above 140 mmHg or a diastolic blood pressure consistently above 90 mmHg. High blood pressure is classified into two categories, primary (or essential) and secondary. Approximately 95% of individuals with hypertension have **primary hypertension,** in which the cause is not apparent. The remaining 5% have **secondary hypertension,** due to endocrine or renal abnormalities. Although primary hypertension has no known direct cause, it is related to a variety of factors, including inactivity, obesity, alcohol intake, and (in sodium-sensitive individuals) salt intake. Regular exercise can play an important role in reducing elevated blood pressure.

CASE STUDY 10.3
Client With Hypertension

Collin F. has a history of hypertension that is currently managed by his physician with beta-blockers. Mr. F. has approached you with a desire to begin an exercise program, because his physician informed him that aerobic exercise will elicit an average reduction of 10 mmHg for both systolic and diastolic blood pressures. Mr. F.'s resting blood pressure is routinely under the 200/110 mmHg level that would contraindicate exercise, and it has never approached a dangerous exaggerated pressor response of 260/115 mmHg during exercise.

Exercise prescription for hypertensive patients follows the general guidelines for the healthy population as summarized in table 2.1. Some considerations must be made based on medications and to avoid hypertensive responses to the exercise itself. Your exercise prescription for Mr. F., following the FITT principle and ACSM guidelines (Franklin 2000; Gordon 1997), is as follows:

Frequency: You recommend three to seven days per week to maximize the benefits of blood pressure reduction from exercise.

Intensity: You decide on an intensity of 40-70% of $\dot{V}O_2$max. Note: the ACSM has changed the basis for cardiorespiratory exercise prescription from % $\dot{V}O_2$max to % $\dot{V}O_2R$ for most situations; however, it still retains the terminology of %$\dot{V}O_2$max for certain special populations (Franklin 2000). Mr. F.'s beta-blocker will attenuate his heart rate by about 30 beats per minute. Therefore, prescribing exercise by target heart rate, especially using methods that estimate the maximal heart rate, may not be appropriate. If stress test data on Mr. F. had been obtained while he was taking his medication, you could use that information to determine a target HR or work rate. In Mr. F.'s case, this information is not

(continued)

Case Study 10.3 *(continued)*

available. Thus, you initially prescribe his intensity at a low level using 11-13 on the RPE scale.

Time: You decide on 30-60 minutes per exercise session.

Type: You recommend large muscle activities for aerobic exercise, such as walking, cycling, or swimming. You may prescribe resistance training later on, preferably using circuit weight training with high repetitions (10-15) and low resistance. You instruct Mr. F. to avoid the Valsalva maneuver during his resistance exercise.

PREGNANCY

Exercise during pregnancy provides many benefits to the woman while entailing few risks to the developing fetus. Benefits to the woman include the same fitness and health benefits available to nonpregnant exercisers. In addition, women who exercise during pregnancy can generally expect a less difficult delivery and a faster return to prepregnancy weight and fitness than nonexercising pregnant women.

Women who exercise during their pregnancies report no increases in adverse effects, such as spontaneous abortions or birth abnormalities, compared with women who are sedentary during pregnancy. However, the American College of Obstetricians and Gynecologists (ACOG) has established contraindications for exercise during pregnancy (Franklin 2000). Therefore, women should obtain a physician's clearance before starting an exercise program during pregnancy, especially if they were sedentary before their pregnancy. Women who have been exercising regularly may continue to participate in their current exercise program, modifying the intensity, duration, and frequency as needed as the pregnancy progresses.

CASE STUDY 10.4
Pregnant Client

Kerri B. is 35 years old and has recently discovered she is pregnant. She is in her first trimester and wants to continue her exercise program. She is referred to you by her physician with permission to continue her current exercise program, provided she reduces her exercise as overall discomfort or specific symptoms dictate. Her current exercise program consists of aerobic and resistance training: she runs three or four times each week for a total of about 12-15 miles, and she exercises all her major muscle groups with resistance training twice a week.

Because Ms. B. has a very active history of exercise before her pregnancy, she should be able to adjust comfortably to an exercise program during her pregnancy. You recommend the following exercise program following ACSM/ACOG guidelines (Franklin 2000):

Frequency: Ms. B. is to continue exercising at least three times per week after her regular exercise routine.

Intensity: Standard guidelines for intensity apply to pregnant women. However, because maximal HR decreases during pregnancy and resting HR increases, target HR calculations are not applicable. Furthermore, although maximal exercise testing during pregnancy has not been reported to have adverse effects, it generally is not recommended and is of limited use. Therefore, you recommend that Ms. B. use ratings of perceived exertion to monitor intensity. A special concern is that she avoid overheating during exercise, especially during the first trimester, when the fetus is most susceptible to heat-induced defects in development. Therefore you instruct Ms. B. not to exercise in hot conditions and to remain properly hydrated.

Time: The duration of the exercise session may require daily adjustments. She should not continue an exercise session to the point of fatigue or exhaustion.

Type: Ms. B. may perform weightbearing aerobic exercise; but you point out that nonweightbearing exercises such as cycling and swimming will minimize the risk of injury, and she can perform them more comfortably—which will facilitate her continuing the exercises in the latter stages of her pregnancy. After the first trimester, she should avoid exercising in the supine position (especially if the exercise is prolonged), because it may result in a reduction in blood flow to the uterus. She should be able to fully resume her prepregnancy exercise routines 4-6 weeks postpartum.

Exercise recommendations during pregnancy for women who do not regularly exercise are similar to those listed previously. However, such individuals may require supervision and should be taught the signs and symptoms that require discontinuing exercise (Franklin 2000).

CHILDREN

Since the advent of television, childhood physical activity levels have been on the decline—a trend that has increased with the widespread use of the computer as an entertainment medium. Childhood obesity is becoming epidemic, along with obesity-related diseases such as type 2 diabetes. Exercise guidelines for children need to emphasize *the enjoyment of physical activity as a lifelong pursuit.* This section provides information regarding exercise recommendations for healthy children ranging in age from 6-17 years, encompassing both preadolescence and adolescence.

Aerobic Exercise

The principal recommendation of the ACSM (as well as the Centers for Disease Control and the U.S. Surgeon General) is that all individuals aged six years and above should engage in at least 30 minutes of moderate physical activity on most, and preferably all, days of the week (Pate et al. 1995; U.S. Department of Health and Human Services 1996). Thus, even very young children should be engaging in regular physical activity. Preadolescents should focus on physically active play rather than on intense, structured, aerobic conditioning. Older children can benefit from vigorous aerobic training by following standard prescription guidelines, although the use of heart rate prescriptions is generally not necessary.

Intensity is not as important as establishing a daily routine of activity. All children can exercise at a variety of intensities and durations; if given the choice, however, most prefer short-term intermittent activities that have a high recreational component. Most children prefer skill-related sports such as tennis, soccer, and basketball to running on a treadmill, and they generally choose outdoor bicycling rather than stationary cycling. Furthermore, children seem to tolerate activities that are repeated and have a short duration with rest periods. The least physiologically tolerable types of activities are ones that are highly anaerobic and last from 10-90 seconds—e.g., running sprints in a fitness class.

Aerobic exercise prescription for all children should focus on keeping the children active, rather than increasing their functional capacity or $\dot{V}O_2$max. Recommended activities are those that require moving the whole body, such as running, swimming, and cycling. Furthermore, because children are involved in a variety of activities throughout the day, it's best if they set aside a specific time for sustained aerobic activities. All these approaches can help maximize the volume of energy expended, which is extremely beneficial in obese children.

One concern about children's aerobic exercise is that their metabolic rate *per unit of body mass* is higher when compared with adults at a given submaximal walking or running speed. Children therefore produce excessive body heat when exercising and have a higher energy expenditure than adults. Yet their immature cardiovascular systems, with low blood flow capacity in the skin, result in reduced capacity for sweating. These factors, combined with a large surface area-to-body mass ratio in children, result in a low tolerance to hot weather and a greater susceptibility to heat stress, especially during continuous activities. The high surface area-to-body mass ratio also accelerates heat loss during exposure to the cold and can increase the risk of hypothermia. In warm weather, it takes children about 10-14 days to acclimate to a hot environment. They should wear loose, lightweight clothing that readily permits air flow, to allow for the evaporation of sweat. When air temperature and humidity levels are high, children should reduce activities that last longer than 30 minutes, and they should be instructed to drink 100-150 ml of fluid every 15-30 minutes, whether or not they feel thirsty. Cold water is more easily absorbed than warm; if a sports drink is consumed instead of water, it should contain no more than 25g of sugar per liter (Bar-Or 1983).

Activities that involve repeated mechanical stress over a long period of time can cause overuse injuries in children. For example, excessive endurance activities can damage epiphyseal growth plates and growth tissues. For these reasons, young runners may be more prone to musculoskeletal problems than adults. Other risks include any sudden change (more than 10% in a week) in the intensity, duration, or frequency of the exercise; musculotendinous imbalances; incorrect biomechanics; and improper footwear / running surfaces.

Resistance Training

Resistance training is appropriate for children, with only a few cautions relative to the guidelines for adults. The ACSM recommends that children not attempt maximal lifts until they reach adolescence, and that they perform resistance training only twice a week (Franklin 2000). In all other aspects, the ACSM guidelines for children's resistance training are the same as those for adults, as summarized in table 2.1. In particular, children should perform at least one set of 8-10 different exercises that work all major muscle groups, with a range of 8-12 repetitions.

A qualified adult should always supervise resistance training by children. Be certain that you teach children (as well as all novice lifters) proper lifting technique. Remember that even large and strong children may still be physiologically immature.

CASE STUDY 10.5
High School Football Player

Billy is a 15-year-old high school sophomore who wants to try out for the football team next fall. He weighs 150 lb and is 5'10" tall. His coach has recommended that he increase his body weight and participate in a resistance training program over the summer to increase his strength and size.

Billy has decided to lift weights at the neighborhood YMCA, where a combination of free weights and circuit training machines are available. Because Billy has never been involved in a structured weightlifting program, you decide to have him begin with the circuit weight machines, exercising all his major muscle groups two times per week on Monday and Thursday. You design the following program for Billy, using a series of weightlifting machines:

Frequency: Twice per week.

Intensity: Weight loads that allow 8-12 repetitions.

Time: Perform 1-2 sets of 8-10 different exercises using the machines. Rest for periods of at least 1-2 minutes between sets and exercises.

Type: Progress along the circuit, training all major muscle groups, beginning with large muscle groups and ending with smaller ones.

(Refer to chapter 6 for a complete description of exercises.)

In addition, you encourage Billy to participate in moderate-intensity aerobic activities for 30 minutes, three times a week. You instruct him not to engage in strenuous or prolonged aerobic conditioning, so that the extra caloric expenditure does not interfere with his desire to gain weight. You also work with him to develop an appropriate nutritional program comprising sufficient total calories as well as quality protein sources.

REFERENCES

1. Bar-Or, O. 1983. *Pediatric Sports Medicine for the Practitioner: From Physiologic Principles to Clinical Applications.* New York: Springer.

2. Franklin, BA, ed. 2000. *ACSM's Guidelines for Exercise Testing and Prescription,* 6th ed., 200-205, 206-210, 217-234. Philadelphia: Lippincott Williams & Wilkins.

3. Gardner, A. 1997. Peripheral vascular disease. In *ACSM's Exercise Management for Persons With Chronic Diseases and Disabilities,* ed. JL Durstine, 64-68. Champaign, IL: Human Kinetics.

4. Gordon, NF. 1997. Hypertension. In *ACSM's Exercise Management for Persons With Chronic Diseases and Disabilities,* ed. JL Durstine, 59-63. Champaign, IL: Human Kinetics.

5. Pate, RR, ed. 1991. *ACSM's Guidelines for Exercise Testing and Prescription,* 4th ed., 73. Philadelphia: Lea & Febiger.

6. Pate, RR, M Pratt, SN Blair, WL Haskell, CA Macera, C Bouchard, D Buchner, W Ettinger, GW Heath, and AC King. 1995. Physical activity and public health. A recommendation from the Centers for Disease Control and Prevention and the American College of Sports Medicine. *J. Am. Med. Assoc.* 273:402-407.

7. U.S. Department of Health and Human Services. 1996. *Physical Activity and Health: A Report of the Surgeon General.* Atlanta, GA: U.S. Department of Health and Human Services, Centers for Disease Control and Prevention, National Center for Chronic Disease Prevention and Health Promotion.

Additional Case Studies With Multiple Choice Questions

Young Adult Client

Marina C. is a 36-year-old nonsmoker who weighs 108 lb and is 5'1" tall. She lifts weights and jogs several times per week. Her father had a heart attack when he was 49 years old, and her mother was diagnosed with breast cancer when she was 58 years old. Ms. C. has recently had a complete fitness evaluation, which included the following: Her resting blood pressure and heart rate are 98/64 mmHg and 68 bpm, respectively. Her lipid profile is total cholesterol of 182 mg·dl⁻¹, LDL cholesterol 118 mg·dl⁻¹, HDL cholesterol 52 mg·dl⁻¹, and fasting glucose is 93 mg·dl⁻¹. Her estimated $\dot{V}O_2$max is 42 ml·min⁻¹·kg⁻¹ (90th percentile). Other fitness measures are 1-RM bench press 85 lb (90th percentile), 44 partial curl-ups (80th percentile) and 31 cm sit-and-reach score on box with 26 cm at foot-line (40th percentile).

1. Ms. C.'s body mass index is

   a. in the "underweight" category

   b. 20.4 kg·m⁻²

   c. 24.6 kg·m⁻²

   d. 29.0 kg·m⁻²

(continued)

Case Study A.1   *(continued)*

2. *Which of the following ACSM risk factors does Ms. C. have?*
    a. obesity
    b. family history
    c. hypercholesterolemia
    d. negative risk factor for high HDL

3. *To which risk stratification category does Ms. C. belong?*
    a. low-risk
    b. moderate-risk
    c. high-risk

4. *If Ms. C. wishes to exercise in your facility, will she need physician clearance first?*
    a. yes, if the exercise is to be vigorous; but no if moderate
    b. yes, if the exercise is to be moderate or vigorous
    c. no, for moderate or vigorous exercise

5. *What would be Ms. C.'s target heart rate at 70% of $\dot{V}O_2R$, using the %HRmax method (hint: see table 3.1)?*
    a. 129 bpm
    b. 155 bpm
    c. 172 bpm
    d. 184 bpm

6. *What would be Ms. C.'s target heart rate at 70% of $\dot{V}O_2R$, using the %HRR method?*
    a. 81 bpm
    b. 116 bpm
    c. 136 bpm
    d. 149 bpm

7. *What would be Ms. C.'s gross oxygen consumption at 70% of $\dot{V}O_2R$?*
    a. 38.5 ml·min^{-1}·kg^{-1}
    b. 30.5 ml·min^{-1}·kg^{-1}
    c. 29.4 ml·min^{-1}·kg^{-1}
    d. 27.0 ml·min^{-1}·kg^{-1}

8. *For indoor aerobic exercise, Ms. C. would like to walk on a treadmill. If she walks at 3.5 mph, what % grade would allow her to exercise at 70% of $\dot{V}O_2R$?*

  a. 8%

  b. 9%

  c. 10%

  d. She cannot walk at 3.5 mph and attain the desired $\dot{V}O_2$ on a treadmill.

9. *What would be Ms. C.'s net caloric expenditure at 70% of $\dot{V}O_2R$?*

  a. 6.6 kcal·min^{-1}

  b. 7.5 kcal·min^{-1}

  c. 9.5 kcal·min^{-1}

  d. 10.3 kcal·min^{-1}

10. *Based on Ms. C.'s fitness assessment, which component of fitness should she most work to improve?*

  a. body composition

  b. aerobic capacity

  c. muscular strength

  d. flexibility

CASE STUDY A.2
Young Adult Client

Heather F. is 43 years old, weighs 142 lb, and is 5'5" tall. She is a former one-pack-a-day cigarette smoker, having quit smoking two years ago. She has a sedentary job, but sometimes takes a 15-minute walk at lunch time. Her father had coronary angioplasty when he was 61 years old. Her resting blood pressure and heart rate are 132/84 mmHg and 78 bpm, respectively. Her lipid profile is total cholesterol of 194 mg·dl^{-1}, LDL 134 mg·dl^{-1}, and HDL 45 mg·dl^{-1}. Fasting glucose is 102 mg·dl^{-1}. Her estimated $\dot{V}O_2$max is 27 ml·min^{-1}·kg^{-1} (20th percentile). Other fitness measures are an estimated body fat (skinfolds) of 28% (40th percentile), 12 modified pushups (50th percentile), 14 partial curl-ups (30th percentile) and 24-cm sit-and-reach score on box with 26 cm at foot line (20th percentile).

(continued)

Case Study A.2 *(continued)*

11. Which of the following ACSM risk factors does Ms. F. have?
    a. obesity
    b. family history
    c. sedentary lifestyle
    d. hypercholesterolemia
    e. both a and b
    f. both c and d

12. To which risk stratification category does Ms. F. belong?
    a. low-risk
    b. moderate-risk
    c. high-risk

13. If Ms. F. wishes to exercise in your facility, will she need physician clearance first?
    a. yes, if the exercise is to be vigorous; but no if moderate
    b. yes, if the exercise is to be moderate or vigorous
    c. no, for moderate or vigorous exercise

14. What would be Ms. F.'s target heart rate at 50% of $\dot{V}O_2R$, using the %HRR method?
    a. 177 bpm
    b. 128 bpm
    c. 99 bpm
    d. 89 bpm

15. What would be Ms. F.'s target workload on a leg cycle ergometer at 50% of $\dot{V}O_2R$?
    a. 50 W
    b. 125 W
    c. 450 kg·m·min^{-1}
    d. 600 kg·m·min^{-1}

16. If Ms. F. is cycling on a Monark bike ergometer at 50 rpm, what resistance setting in kg would place her at 50% of $\dot{V}O_2R$?
    a. 0.5 kg
    b. 1.0 kg
    c. 1.5 kg
    d. 2.0 kg

17. *For improving cardiorespiratory fitness, what frequency of exercise should you recommend for Ms. F.?*

    a. 2-3 times per week

    b. 3-5 times per week

    c. 4-6 times per week

    d. 5-7 times per week

18. *For improving muscular strength and muscular endurance, what repetition range for resistance exercise should you recommend for Ms. F.?*

    a. 4-6

    b. 6-10

    c. 8-12

    d. 10-15

19. *For improving muscular fitness, what frequency of exercise should you recommend for Ms. F.?*

    a. 2-3 times per week

    b. 3-5 times per week

    c. 4-6 times per week

    d. 5-7 times per week

20. *When she performs flexibility exercises, which of the following would be contraindicated for Ms. F?*

    a. bouncing to achieve a greater stretch

    b. curving the upper body downward while performing a hamstring stretch

    c. performing a "hurdler's" stretch with the opposite knee bent rearwards

    d. all of the above

CASE STUDY A.3
Weight Loss Client

Frank G. is 27 years old, weighs 212 lb and is 5'8" tall. He is a sedentary nonsmoker. His father was diagnosed with type 2 diabetes at 51 years of age, and his mother had a heart attack when she was 62. His resting blood pressure and heart rate are 146/94

(continued)

Case Study A.3 *(continued)*

mmHg and 84 bpm, respectively. His lipid profile is total choles-terol of 234 mg·dl⁻¹, LDL 142 mg·dl⁻¹, and HDL 46 mg·dl⁻¹. Fasting glucose is 106 mg·dl⁻¹. After complaining of chest pain during a softball game, he was given a stress test. His measured $\dot{V}O_2$max was 24 ml·min⁻¹·kg⁻¹ (< 10th percentile). His maximal heart rate was 198 bpm. There were no signs or symptoms of heart disease, and his physician has cleared him for exercise. His body fat has been measured by hydrostatic weighing as 35% (< 10th percentile).

21. *In what category is Mr. G.'s body mass index?*
   a. class II obesity
   b. class I obesity
   c. overweight
   d. normal

22. *How many ACSM risk factors does Mr. G. have?*
   a. 4
   b. 5
   c. 6
   d. 7

23. *What is Mr. G.'s current lean body weight?*
   a. 74 lb
   b. 118 lb
   c. 127 lb
   d. 138 lb

24. *What would Mr. G. weigh at 20% body fat, assuming no change in his lean body mass?*
   a. 158 lb
   b. 172 lb
   c. 180 lb
   d. 197 lb

25. *How long should Mr. G. take to reach his goal weight at 20% body fat?*
   a. 20 to 40 weeks
   b. 6 months to a year

c. one to two years

d. 15 to 30 weeks

26. What would be Mr. G.'s target heart rate at 50% of $\dot{V}O_2R$, using the %HRR method?

a. 139 bpm

b. 141 bpm

c. 151 bpm

d. 163 bpm

27. What walking speed on flat ground would place Mr. G. at 50% of $\dot{V}O_2R$?

a. 2.5 mph

b. 2.8 mph

c. 3.4 mph

d. 3.8 mph

28. What work rate on a leg cycle ergometer would place Mr. G. at 50% of $\dot{V}O_2R$?

a. 100 W

b. 75 W

c. 400 kg·m·min^{-1}

d. 360 kg·m·min^{-1}

29. What would be Mr. G.'s net caloric expenditure at 50% of $\dot{V}O_2R$?

a. 5.0 kcal·min^{-1}

b. 6.6 kcal·min^{-1}

c. 7.5 kcal·min^{-1}

d. 9.5 kcal·min^{-1}

30. If Mr. G. walks every day, how many minutes per day would be required for him to lose $\frac{1}{2}$ lb of fat each week through the exercise alone?

a. 38 minutes

b. 45 minutes

c. 50 minutes

d. 60 minutes

> ## CASE STUDY A.4
> ### *Older Adult Client*

Arthur B. is 71 years old, weighs 176 lb, and is 5'10" tall. He is a pipe smoker. He likes to play golf, but uses a cart. His sister had bypass surgery when she was 64 years old. His resting blood pressure and heart rate are 128/82 mmHg and 90 bpm, respectively. His lipid profile is total cholesterol of 204 mg·dl⁻¹, LDL 126 mg·dl⁻¹, and HDL 39 mg·dl⁻¹. Fasting glucose is 94 mg·dl⁻¹. His estimated $\dot{V}O_2$max is 18 ml·min⁻¹·kg⁻¹ (< 10th percentile). Other fitness measures are six pushups (30th percentile), nine partial curl-ups (40th percentile), and 19-cm sit-and-reach score on box with 26 cm at foot line (40th percentile). He has moderate to severe arthritis in his knees.

31. *Which of the following ACSM risk factors does Mr. B. have?*
    a. family history
    b. sedentary lifestyle
    c. obesity
    d. hypercholesterolemia
    e. a and b
    f. all of the above

32. *To which risk stratification category does Mr. B. belong?*
    a. low-risk
    b. moderate-risk
    c. high-risk

33. *To improve his muscular strength and muscular endurance, how many different resistance training exercises should Mr. B. perform?*
    a. 3-4
    b. 5-6
    c. 6-8
    d. 8-10

34. *To improve his muscular strength and muscular endurance, what repetition range should Mr. B. perform according to the ACSM?*
    a. 6-8
    b. 8-12

c. 10-15

d. 12-15

35. *For which of the following reasons is a target heart rate likely to be inaccurate in Mr. B.'s case?*

   a. The elderly do not have a linear response of heart rate to workload.

   b. In the elderly, %HRR and %$\dot{V}O_2R$ are not closely related.

   c. You don't know Mr. B.'s true maximum HR.

   d. Arthritis affects the HR response to exercise.

36. *If you were to prescribe Mr. B. a target HR, what would it be at 40% of $\dot{V}O_2R$ using the %HRmax method (hint: see table 3.1)?*

   a. 95 bpm

   b. 114 bpm

   c. 122 bpm

   d. 141 bpm

37. *If you were to prescribe Mr. B. a target HR, what would it be at 40% of $\dot{V}O_2R$ using the %HRR method?*

   a. 95 bpm

   b. 114 bpm

   c. 122 bpm

   d. 141 bpm

38. *Which mode of cardiorespiratory exercise would be preferred for Mr. B.?*

   a. jogging

   b. bench stepping

   c. water aerobics

   d. a or b

39. *What workload on an arm ergometer would place Mr. B. at 40% of $\dot{V}O_2R$?*

   a. 26 W

   b. 32 W

   c. 250 kg·m·min^{-1}

   d. 360 kg·m·min^{-1} *(continued)*

Case Study A.4 *(continued)*

40. What RPE range would approximate 40-60% of $\dot{V}O_2R$ for Mr. B?
   a. 12-14
   b. 13-15
   c. 14-16
   d. 15-17

CASE STUDY A.5
Client With Myocardial Infarction

Andy M. is a sedentary 45-year-old smoker who weighs 245 lb and is 5′10″ tall. He was recently admitted to the hospital complaining of chest pain. His cardiac blood enzymes were elevated along with his ST-segments, confirming a myocardial infarction in progress. Mr. M. was rushed to the catheterization lab where it was determined that his left anterior descending artery was blocked at the proximal end. He underwent percutaneous transluminal coronary angioplasty (PTCA), which was successful. His ejection fraction is 55%. Two weeks have passed and Mr. M. is ready to begin your Phase II cardiac rehabilitation program. A recent nonmaximal stress test following the Bruce protocol was terminated at 85% of the predicted maximum heart rate and revealed the following data:

Resting HR: 80 bpm

Resting BP: 142/90 mmHg

Peak HR: 145 bpm (test terminated at ~85% of age-estimated HRmax)

Peak BP: 182/96 mmHg

Test terminated at 8:00 minutes into Bruce protocol (3.4 mph, 14% grade)

Medications: Aspirin, Cardizem

Other information from Mr. M.'s chart indicated a lipid profile with a total cholesterol of 250 mg·dl⁻¹, LDL 160 mg·dl⁻¹, and HDL 35 mg·dl⁻¹. His father died of a heart attack at age 56. Mr. M. is currently working as a salesman for a large paper company and has no physically active recreational pursuits.

41. *How many risk factors does Mr. M. have for coronary artery disease?*
   a. 2
   b. 3
   c. 4
   d. 5

42. *What is Mr. M.'s body mass index?*
   a. 30.3 kg·m⁻²
   b. 35.1 kg·m⁻²
   c. 42.6 kg·m⁻²

43. *In which ACSM risk stratification category does Mr. M. belong?*
   a. low-risk
   b. moderate-risk
   c. high-risk

44. *Based on the above stress test information, at approximately what gross oxygen consumption was the stress test stopped?*
   a. 30.7 ml·min⁻¹·kg⁻¹
   b. 35.5 ml·min⁻¹·kg⁻¹
   c. 42.9 ml·min⁻¹·kg⁻¹
   d. 54.0 ml·min⁻¹·kg⁻¹

45. *Approximately how many kilocalories per minute (gross) was Mr. M. expending during the final stage of his treadmill test?*
   a. 10
   b. 15
   c. 20
   d. 25

46. *Calculate a target heart rate for Mr. M. at 60% and 80% of $\dot{V}O_2R$, using the %HRR method.*
   a. 140-182 bpm
   b. 137-156 bpm
   c. 155-183 bpm
   d. 142-156 bpm

(continued)

Case Study A.5 *(continued)*

47. *What would be Mr. M.'s target heart rate at 70% of V̇O₂R using the %HRmax method? (hint: see table 3.1)*
    a. 120 bpm
    b. 135 bpm
    c. 147 bpm
    d. 169 bpm

48. *You want to prescribe Mr. M. a weight-training program when he completes Phase II. Based on the ACSM guidelines, what should the frequency and intensity be?*
    a. 2-3 days per week, 10-15 rep range
    b. 5-6 days per week, 80% of the 1-RM
    c. 7 days per week as tolerated
    d. 2 days per week, light weight and very high reps (> 15)

49. *Traditionally, Mr. M.'s phase II rehabilitation is expected to last for how long?*
    a. 6 weeks
    b. 8 weeks
    c. 12 weeks
    d. 24 months

50. *At the conclusion of his phase II program, you wish to re-evaluate his aerobic fitness. Which of the following tests can you perform without the presence of a physician?*
    a. submaximal
    b. maximal
    c. either submaximal or maximal
    d. neither submaximal nor maximal

CASE STUDY A.6
Client With Pacemaker

John P. is a 50-year-old sedentary male who was seen by his physician with the primary complaint of tiredness. His weight and height are 170 lb and 5'9". He is a nonsmoker, with no history of heart disease in his family. A blood lipid profile reported a total cholesterol level of 189 mg·dl⁻¹, HDL 36 mg·dl⁻¹, and LDL 135 mg·dl⁻¹. A resting ECG determined a bradycardic heart rate. Mr. P. was referred to a cardiologist who specialized in the electrophysiology of the heart. He diagnosed chronotropic incompetence, with adequate sinus node function and high-grade AV block. Therefore, it was recommended that Mr. P. receive a DDDR pacemaker so that AV synchrony, rate responsiveness, and atrial tracking would occur during activity. Three weeks following the implantation of the pacemaker, he underwent a maximal exercise test before entering your Phase II cardiac rehabilitation program, and his estimated $\dot{V}O_2$max was 35 ml·min⁻¹·kg⁻¹. His resting heart rate and blood pressure were 70 bpm and 110/70 mmHg. Peak heart rate and blood pressure were 160 bpm and 172/80 mmHg.

51. *How many coronary artery disease risk factors (do not include his pacemaker) does Mr. P. have?*
    a. 1
    b. 2
    c. 3
    d. 4

52. *What is Mr. P.'s body mass index?*
    a. 20 kg·m⁻²
    b. 25 kg·m⁻²
    c. 30 kg·m⁻²
    d. 42 kg·m⁻²

53. *Based on Mr. P.'s BMI, what classification of disease risk is he in?*
    a. underweight
    b. normal
    c. overweight
    d. obesity

54. *What would be Mr. P.'s target heart rate at 70% of $\dot{V}O_2R$, using the %HRR method?*
    a. 119 bpm
    b. 133 bpm
    c. 140 bpm
    d. 148 bpm

(continued)

Case Study A.6   *(continued)*

55. *To reach his target HR, Mr. P. must walk 3.0 mph at a grade of 10%. What is his estimated gross $\dot{V}O_2$ at this speed and grade?*

    a. 15 ml·min⁻¹·kg⁻¹

    b. 20 ml·min⁻¹·kg⁻¹

    c. 26 ml·min⁻¹·kg⁻¹

    d. 29 ml·min⁻¹·kg⁻¹

56. *How many gross kilocalories per minute would Mr. P. be expending at his peak $\dot{V}O_2$?*

    a. 13.5

    b. 15

    c. 23

    d. There is not enough information to calculate his caloric expenditure.

57. *To exercise at 60% of $\dot{V}O_2R$ on an 8″ high bench, what stepping rate would he need to use?*

    a. 15 steps·min⁻¹

    b. 28 steps·min⁻¹

    c. 30 steps·min⁻¹

    d. 42 steps·min⁻¹

58. *Mr. P. has expressed an interest in using a stationary bicycle. What work rate should you set to achieve 70% of $\dot{V}O_2R$?*

    a. 100 W

    b. 130 W

    c. 150 W

    d. 200 W

59. *Mr. P. wants to begin a very light resistance training program and range-of-motion exercises to strengthen his upper body. When should he be able to begin?*

    a. immediately after implantation

    b. 1 week after implantation

    c. 2-3 weeks after implantation

    d. 1 month after implantation

60. *How often should Mr. P.'s resistance training and range-of-motion exercises be performed?*
   a. 1 day per week
   b. 2-3 days per week
   c. 4 days per week
   d. Resistance training and range-of-motion exercises should not be performed during the same week.

CASE STUDY A.7
Client With Type 1 Diabetes

Alejandro R. is a 32-year-old who was diagnosed with type 1 diabetes at the age of 10. His treatment consists of twice-daily injections of both short-acting and intermediate-acting insulin. He weighs 143 lb and is 5'7" tall. His most recent fasting blood test results were total cholesterol of 221 mg·dl^{-1}, LDL 140 mg·dl^{-1}, and HDL 42 mg·dl^{-1}. Fasting glucose was 123 mg·dl^{-1}. His resting blood pressure and heart rate are 124/82 mmHg and 76 bpm, respectively. He has recently tried jogging to "get in better shape," but has experienced several bouts of hypoglycemia. He visited his physician, who has referred him to you for a fitness evaluation and exercise prescription. Results of his fitness evaluation include an estimated $\dot{V}O_2$max of 39 ml·min^{-1}·kg^{-1} (40th percentile), an estimated body fat (skinfolds) of 20% (40th percentile), 22 push-ups (60th percentile), 18 partial curl-ups (~30th percentile), and 18-cm sit-and-reach score on box with 26 cm at foot line (10th percentile).

61. *To which ACSM risk category does Mr. R. belong?*
   a. low-risk
   b. moderate-risk
   c. high-risk

62. *What should be Mr. R.'s first step in adjusting his routine to avoid exercise-induced hypoglycemia?*
   a. Increase insulin dosage before exercise.
   b. Decrease insulin dosage before exercise.
   c. Consume extra carbohydrates throughout the day.
   d. Reduce carbohydrate consumption before exercise.

(continued)

Case Study A.7   *(continued)*

63. *At what frequency should Mr. R. begin his aerobic training program?*

    a. twice per week

    b. 3 times per week

    c. 5 times per week

    d. every day

64. *At what duration should Mr. R. begin his aerobic training program?*

    a. 10-20 min

    b. 20-30 min

    c. 30-40 min

    d. 50-60 min

65. *Which of the following workloads would place Mr. R. at 60% of $\dot{V}O_2R$?*

    a. jogging at 9.7 mph

    b. walking at 3 mph up a 4% grade

    c. stationary biking at 150 W

    d. stepping 26 times per minute on a 10" bench

66. *What would be Mr. R.'s target HR at 60% of $\dot{V}O_2R$, using the %HRR method?*

    a. 113 bpm

    b. 123 bpm

    c. 133 bpm

    d. 143 bpm

67. *Mr. R. measures his blood glucose a few minutes before a planned exercise session and records a value of 85 mg·dl^{-1}. What should he do?*

    a. Remeasure it, as that can't be correct.

    b. Cancel the exercise session.

    c. Eat 20-30 g of carbohydrates, remeasure after 15 min, exercise if then above 100 mg·dl^{-1}.

    d. Begin exercise.

68. Mr. R. measures his blood glucose a few minutes before a planned exercise session and records a value of 260 mg·dl⁻¹. What should he do?

   a. Begin exercise.

   b. Cancel exercise.

   c. Eat 20-30 g of carbohydrates and then exercise.

   d. Check for urinary ketones; if present, cancel exercise.

69. During an exercise session, Mr. R. experiences weakness and lightheadedness. What should he do?

   a. Call 911.

   b. Eat a fast-acting source of sugar to relieve the symptoms.

   c. Lie down and rest until the symptoms go away.

   d. Continue exercising until the symptoms go away.

70. At what repetition range should Mr. R. be performing resistance training?

   a. 8-12

   b. 10-15

   c. 15-20

   d. He should not be doing resistance training.

CASE STUDY A.8
Client With Type 2 Diabetes

William P. is 62 years old and was diagnosed with type 2 diabetes last month. He has been placed on oral hypoglycemic therapy, has seen a nutritionist about improving his diet, and has now been referred to you for an exercise program. A stress test showed that his $\dot{V}O_2$max is 18 ml·min⁻¹·kg⁻¹ (< 10th percentile); his maximal heart rate is 166 bpm. There were no signs or symptoms of heart disease. He weighs 320 lb and is 5'11" tall. His blood test showed a total cholesterol of 284 mg·dl⁻¹, LDL 146 mg·dl⁻¹, and HDL 37 mg·dl⁻¹. Fasting glucose is 184 mg·dl⁻¹. His resting blood pressure and heart rate are 124/82 mmHg and 76 bpm, respectively.

(continued)

Case Study A.8   *(continued)*

71. *In what category is Mr. P.'s body mass index?*
    a. overweight
    b. class I obesity
    c. class II obesity
    d. class III obesity

72. *What would be Mr. P.'s target weight at a BMI of 25 kg·m⁻²?*
    a. 179 lb
    b. 196 lb
    c. 218 lb
    d. 242 lb

73. *What intensity range should Mr. P. be initially prescribed?*
    a. 40-60% $\dot{V}O_2R$
    b. 50-70% $\dot{V}O_2R$
    c. 50-85% $\dot{V}O_2R$
    d. 60-80% $\dot{V}O_2R$

74. *After he has progressed through several weeks of aerobic exercise training, what frequency and duration should Mr. P. be prescribed?*
    a. 20-30 min, 3-5 times per week
    b. 20-30 min, 5-7 times per week
    c. 50-60 min, 3-5 times per week
    d. 50-60 min, 5-7 times per week

75. *If you prescribed a target heart rate at 50% of $\dot{V}O_2R$, what would that be using the %HRR method?*
    a. 102 bpm
    b. 117 bpm
    c. 121 bpm
    d. 132 bpm

76. *What walking speed should Mr. P. be able to maintain on a flat treadmill, assuming 50% of $\dot{V}O_2R$ as the target intensity?*
    a. 2.1 mph
    b. 2.7 mph
    c. 3.2 mph
    d. 3.5 mph

77. What total duration of exercise at 50% of $\dot{V}O_2R$ would Mr. P. need to accumulate in order to lose one lb of fat from the exercise alone?

    a. 4.5 hours

    b. 7.5 hours

    c. 11 hours

    d. 14 hours

78. Prior to one particular exercise session, Mr. P. measures his blood glucose and records a value of 226 $mg \cdot dl^{-1}$. What should he do?

    a. Begin exercise.

    b. Cancel the exercise.

    c. Wait 15 minutes and remeasure.

    d. Check for urinary ketones; if present, cancel exercise.

79. Prior to one particular exercise session, Mr. P. recorded a blood glucose of 176 $mg \cdot dl^{-1}$. Immediately after that exercise session he records a value of 124 $mg \cdot dl^{-1}$. What should he do?

    a. Eat a source of fast-acting sugar.

    b. Go about his day, but be aware of possible hypoglycemia.

    c. Make an immediate appointment with his physician.

    d. Drink a glass of water, wait 15 minutes, and remeasure.

80. Nine months after beginning his exercise and diet program, Mr. P. has lost 52 lb. He has started to experience hypoglycemia during his exercise sessions. What is the best choice for handling this new situation?

    a. Increase his consumption of total daily calories.

    b. Consume 20-30 g of carbohydrates before each exercise bout.

    c. Consult his physician about reducing his hypoglycemic medication.

    d. Ignore the hypoglycemia until he is at his goal weight.

CASE STUDY A.9
Client With Peripheral Vascular Disease

Miguel R. is a 65-year-old sedentary smoker who weighs 234 lb and is 6'3" tall. Lately, Mr. R. has noticed that when he walks, he experiences a burning, tight sensation in his calf muscles. After bringing this to his physician's attention, he was diagnosed with peripheral vascular disease. Due to a high association of cardio-vascular disease and stroke in patients with PVD, Mr. R.'s physician decided to do a treadmill test to evaluate his blood pressure and heart rate during activity. The treadmill test was prematurely stopped due to ischemic leg pain. Therefore, the physician decided to repeat the test using a stationary cycle ergometer. Mr. R. reached a maximal work rate of 200 watts with no signs or symptoms of heart disease. His resting heart rate and blood pressure were 80 bpm and 150/90 mmHg. His peak heart rate and blood pressure were 152 bpm and 250/110 mmHg. A blood lipid profile reported a total cholesterol level of 189 mg·dl^{-1}, HDL 40 mg·dl^{-1}, and LDL 120 mg·dl^{-1}. Mr. R. was prescribed a beta-blocker to treat his high blood pressure and Pentoxifylline for his PVD. He was then referred to you for exercise in your phase III cardiac rehabilitation program.

81. *Based on the above information, what risk factors does Mr. R. have for coronary artery disease?*
    a. sedentary behavior, cigarette smoking, hypertension
    b. hypercholesterolemia
    c. obesity
    d. a and b
    e. a and c

82. *To which risk stratification category does Mr. R. belong?*
    a. low-risk
    b. moderate-risk
    c. high-risk

83. *What ankle-to-arm index for systolic blood pressure is typical of patients with severe PVD?*
    a. 1.1 or higher
    b. 1.0-1.1

c. 0.91-1.0
d. < 0.90

84. *Which modality of exercise would be the most beneficial for improving Mr. R.'s tolerance to leg pain?*
    a. weightbearing exercise
    b. swimming
    c. resistance training
    d. cycling

85. *If Mr. R. stops a walking session due to leg pain, what should you do to extend his exercise session and improve his cardiovascular health?*
    a. Encourage him to run.
    b. Have him seek motivational counseling.
    c. Include nonweightbearing exercises until the leg pain subsides.
    d. Prescribe isometric leg lifts.

86. *When prescribing exercise intensity for Mr. R. using the claudication scale, what grade should be used?*
    a. 1
    b. 2
    c. 3
    d. 4

87. *What is Mr. R.'s estimated gross $\dot{V}O_2max$ from his stationary cycle test?*
    a. 20 ml·min^{-1}·kg^{-1}
    b. 27.3 ml·min^{-1}·kg^{-1}
    c. 30.2 ml·min^{-1}·kg^{-1}
    d. 35 ml·min^{-1}·kg^{-1}

88. *Approximately how many net kilocalories per minute was Mr. R. expending at this work rate?*
    a. 12.7
    b. 14.5
    c. 20.2
    d. 28.7

(continued)

Case Study A.9   *(continued)*

89. *Based on Mr. R.'s stationary cycle test, what would be his target work rate at 50% of* $\dot{V}O_2R$?

    a. 83 W

    b. 100 W

    c. 115 W

    d. 122 W

90. *What effect would the beta-blocker have on Mr. R.'s exercise prescription?*

    a. attenuates his target heart rate

    b. may decrease time to claudication

    c. has no effect

    d. a and b

CASE STUDY A.10
Pregnant Client

Sarah D. is a 24-year-old sedentary woman who has just learned that she is pregnant for the first time. She has heard that exercise can help her during her pregnancy and delivery, so she has come to your fitness facility to start an exercise program.

91. *Which of the following is true concerning Ms. D.'s participation in an exercise program according to ACOG/ACSM guidelines?*

    a. She should obtain physician clearance before beginning.

    b. If you screen her in your facility and she meets low- or moderate-risk criteria, she can begin the program without physician clearance.

    c. At her age, she can begin right away without any screening or clearance.

92. *Once Ms. D. has properly begun her exercise program, which weightlifting exercises should she avoid after the first trimester?*

    a. flat bench press

    b. supine leg press

    c. squats

    d. a and b

93. *In which trimester is it most important to have adequate hydration, and to wear appropriate clothing for heat dissipation?*
    a. first
    b. second
    c. third
    d. they are all equally important

94. *Which of the following statements about exercise and pregnancy is true?*
    a. Healthy pregnant women do not need to limit their exercise for fear of adverse effects.
    b. Spontaneous abortion, preterm labor, and birth abnormalities are more likely in women who exercise during pregnancy.
    c. Strenuous exercise during pregnancy may result in babies with lighter birth weights.
    d. a and c

95. *Maximal exercise testing during pregnancy*
    a. is recommended to determine exercise intensity
    b. is rarely done and generally not recommended
    c. is commonly used to establish $\dot{V}O_2$max during pregnancy
    d. will result in sudden death to the mother

96. *During pregnancy, how should aerobic exercise intensity be determined?*
    a. $\%\dot{V}O_2R$
    b. rating of perceived exertion
    c. %HRR
    d. $\%\dot{V}O_2$max

97. *Most women can return to their prepregnancy exercise routines within what time frame?*
    a. 0-2 weeks postpartum
    b. 2-4 weeks postpartum
    c. 4-6 weeks postpartum
    d. 6-8 weeks postpartum

(continued)

Case Study A.10   *(continued)*

98. *Which of the following benefits can Ms. D. expect from exercising during her pregnancy?*

    a. easier delivery

    b. improved cardiovascular and muscular fitness

    c. more rapid return to prepregnancy weight

    d. all of the above

99. *Why is prescribing exercise intensity via a target heart rate during pregnancy not recommended?*

    a. There are chronotropic alterations during pregnancy that would affect the calculated value for the target heart rate.

    b. Heart rate is too irregular to monitor during pregnancy.

    c. Heart rate and $\dot{V}O_2$ are not linearly related during pregnancy.

    d. The fetal heart rate interferes with measurement of the maternal heart rate.

100. *In order to avoid injury during the latter stages of pregnancy, what should Ms. D. do?*

    a. Stop all exercise during the third trimester.

    b. Never exercise above a heart rate of 140 bpm.

    c. Substitute nonweightbearing exercises for weightbearing exercises.

    d. Exercise only in the early morning.

Answers to Questions

Case Study A.1: 1 b [calculate BMI as lb times 703 divided by in^2], 2 b [father had MI before age 55; see table 1.1], 3 a [young, only one risk factor; see table 1.1], 4 c [low-risk does not need physician clearance; see table 1.1], 5 b [estimate HRmax as 220 – age; multiply by factor in table 3.1], 6 d [target HR = (fractional intensity)(HRmax – HRrest) + HRrest], 7 b [target $\dot{V}O_2$ = (fractional intensity)($\dot{V}O_2$max – 3.5) + 3.5], 8 c [calculate speed in m·min^{-1} as mph × 26.8; solve for grade in the following equation: $\dot{V}O_2$ during walking = 3.5 + 0.1(speed) + 1.8(speed)(fractional grade)], 9 a [net $\dot{V}O_2$ = gross $\dot{V}O_2$ – 3.5; calculate body mass in kg as lb / 2.2; convert $\dot{V}O_2$ in ml·min^{-1}·kg^{-1} to L·min^{-1};

multiply $\dot{V}O_2$ in $L \cdot min^{-1}$ by 5 to attain $kcal \cdot min^{-1}$], 10 d [sit-and-reach score is only at 40th percentile]

Case Study A.2: 11 f [accumulates less than 30 min of moderate exercise most days of the week; LDL cholesterol is > 130 $mg \cdot dl^{-1}$; see table 1.1], 12 b [two risk factors; see table 1.1], 13 a [moderate-risk need physician clearance for vigorous, but not moderate, exercise; see table 1.1], 14 b [estimate HRmax as 220 – age; target HR = (fractional intensity)(HRmax – HRrest) + HRrest], 15 a [target $\dot{V}O_2$ = (fractional intensity)($\dot{V}O_2$max – 3.5) + 3.5; calculate body mass in kg as lb/2.2; solve for workload in the following equation: $\dot{V}O_2$ during leg cycling = 7 + 1.8(workload)/(body mass); calculate power in W as workload in $kg \cdot m \cdot min^{-1}$ divided by 6], 16 b [solve for resistance setting in the following equation: workload = (resistance setting)(6 m)(rpm)], 17 b [see table 2.1], 18 c [see table 2.1], 19 a [see table 2.1], 20 d [static is preferred over ballistic; spine should remain in neutral position; excessive torsion at knee]

Case Study A.3: 21 b [calculate BMI as lb times 703 divided by in^2; see table 1.2], 22 b [obesity, sedentary behavior, maternal MI prior to 65 years of age, hypertension, LDL chol > 130 $mg \cdot dl^{-1}$; see table 1.1], 23 d [fat weight = (% fat)(total body weight); lean body weight = total body weight – fat weight], 24 b [desired weight = (current weight)(1 – current % fat)/(1 – desired % fat); i.e., desired weight = LBW/(desired % lean)], 25 a [recommended rate of fat loss is 1-2 lb per week], 26 b [target HR = (fractional intensity)(HRmax – HRrest) + HRrest; note: use known HRmax], 27 d [target $\dot{V}O_2$ = (fractional intensity)($\dot{V}O_2$max – 3.5) + 3.5; solve for walking speed in following equation: $\dot{V}O_2$ during walking = 3.5 + 0.1(speed) + 1.8(speed)(fractional grade); note: since grade is zero, last term drops out; calculate speed in mph as $m \cdot min^{-1}$ divided by 26.8], 28 d [calculate body mass in kg as lb/2.2; solve for workload in the following equation: $\dot{V}O_2$ during leg cycling = 7 + 1.8(workload)/(body mass)], 29 a [net $\dot{V}O_2$ = gross $\dot{V}O_2$ – 3.5; convert $\dot{V}O_2$ in $ml \cdot min^{-1} \cdot kg^{-1}$ to $L \cdot min^{-1}$; multiply $\dot{V}O_2$ in $L \cdot min^{-1}$ by 5 to attain $kcal \cdot min^{-1}$], 30 c [1 lb of fat contains 3500 kcal; divide one half this value by the net caloric expenditure rate to obtain total minutes needed; divide this value by 7, for daily time required]

Case Study A.4: 31 e [sister with bypass surgery prior to age of 65; sedentary; even though total cholesterol is high, LDL is not; see table 1.1], 32 b [two risk factors, also age; see table 1.1], 33 d [see table 2.1], 34 c [ACSM recommends higher repetition range for the elderly], 35 c [220 – age is a rough estimate, especially in the elderly], 36 a [estimate

HRmax as 220 – age; multiply by factor in table 3.1], 37 b [target HR = (fractional intensity)(HRmax – HRrest) + HRrest], 38 c [low impact for moderate to severe arthritis], 39 a [target $\dot{V}O_2$ = (fractional intensity) ($\dot{V}O_2$max – 3.5) + 3.5; calculate body mass in kg as lb/2.2; solve for workload in the following equation: $\dot{V}O_2$ for arm cycling = 3.5 + 3(workload)/(body mass); calculate power in W as workload in kg·m·min^{-1} divided by 6], 40 a [see table 3.1]

Case Study A.5: 41 d [sedentary, cigarette smoker, obesity based on BMI, hypertension, LDL cholesterol > 130 mg·dl^{-1}; see table 1.1], 42 b [calculate BMI as lb times 703 divided by in^2], 43 c [cardiac disease; see table 1.1], 44 b [calculate speed in m·min^{-1} as mph × 26.8; $\dot{V}O_2$ during walking = 3.5 + 0.1(speed) + 1.8(speed)(fractional grade)], 45 c [calculate body mass in kg as lb/2.2; convert $\dot{V}O_2$ in ml·min^{-1}·kg^{-1} to L·min^{-1}; multiply $\dot{V}O_2$ in L·min^{-1} by 5 to attain kcal·min^{-1}], 46 b [estimate HRmax as 220 – age, since stress test did not go to maximum; target HR = (fractional intensity)(HRmax – HRrest) + HRrest], 47 c [multiply estimated HRmax by factor in table 3.1], 48 a [10-15 rep range is recommended by ACSM for cardiac patients], 49 c [in some cases, phase II programs are reduced in length for low-risk clients, or as a result of insurance reimbursement; however, the standard length has been 12 weeks], 50 d [cardiovascular testing of high-risk clients must be supervised by a physician; see table 1.1]

Case Study A.6: 51 b [sedentary, LDL cholesterol > 130 mg·dl^{-1}; see table 1.1], 52 b [calculate BMI as lb times 703 divided by in^2], 53 c [see table 1.2], 54 b [use reported HRmax; target HR = (fractional intensity)(HRmax – HRrest) + HRrest], 55 c [calculate speed in m·min^{-1} as mph × 26.8; $\dot{V}O_2$ during walking = 3.5 + 0.1(speed) + 1.8(speed)(fractional grade)], 56 a [calculate body mass in kg as lb/2.2; convert $\dot{V}O_2$max in ml·min^{-1}·kg^{-1} to L·min^{-1}; multiply $\dot{V}O_2$ in L·min^{-1} by 5 to attain kcal·min^{-1}], 57 b [target $\dot{V}O_2$ = (fractional intensity)($\dot{V}O_2$max – 3.5) + 3.5; calculate bench height in m as inches times 0.0254; solve for stepping rate using the following equation: $\dot{V}O_2$ during stepping = 3.5 + 0.2(stepping rate) + 2.4(stepping rate)(step height)], 58 b [target $\dot{V}O_2$ = (fractional intensity)($\dot{V}O_2$max – 3.5) + 3.5; calculate body mass in kg as lb/2.2; solve for workload in the following equation: $\dot{V}O_2$ during leg cycling = 7 + 1.8(workload)/(body mass); calculate power in W as workload in kg·m·min^{-1} divided by 6], 59 c [this delay is needed for surgical recovery], 60 b [see table 2.1]

Case Study A.7: 61 c [metabolic disease; see table 1.1], 62 b [see table 9.2], 63 b [see table 2.1], 64 b [see table 2.1], 65 d [target $\dot{V}O_2$ = (frac-

tional intensity)($\dot{V}O_2$max – 3.5) + 3.5; select appropriate equations
from table 4.1], 66 d [estimate HRmax as 220 – age; target HR =
(fractional intensity)(HRmax – HRrest) + HRrest], 67 c [see table 9.3],
68 d [see table 9.3], 69 b [see table 9.2], 70 a [see table 2.1]

Case Study A.8: 71 d [calculate BMI as lb times 703 divided by in²; see
table 1.2], 72 a [enter current height and desired BMI into BMI equation and solve for weight], 73 a [low end of ACSM intensity range is
used for type 2 diabetics and/or those needing weight loss], 74 d
[duration and frequency need to be high to maximize caloric expendi-
ture], 75 c [use known HRmax; target HR = (fractional
intensity)(HRmax – HRrest) + HRrest], 76 b [target $\dot{V}O_2$ = (fractional
intensity)($\dot{V}O_2$max – 3.5) + 3.5; solve for walking speed in following
equation: $\dot{V}O_2$ during walking = 3.5 + 0.1(speed) +
1.8(speed)(fractional grade); note: since grade is zero, last term drops
out; calculate speed in mph as m·min⁻¹ divided by 26.8], 77 c [calculate
body mass in kg as lb/2.2; net $\dot{V}O_2$ = gross $\dot{V}O_2$ – 3.5; convert $\dot{V}O_2$ in
ml·min⁻¹·kg⁻¹ to L·min⁻¹; multiply $\dot{V}O_2$ in L·min⁻¹ by 5 to attain kcal·min⁻¹;
since 1 lb of fat contains 3500 kcal, divide this value by the net caloric
expenditure rate to obtain total minutes needed, convert to hours], 78
a [see table 9.3], 79 b [see table 9.2], 80 c [exercise training improves
insulin sensitivity, and patients may need to reduce hypoglycemic
medications]

Case Study A.9: 81 a [see table 1.1; BMI of 29.2 kg·m⁻² is "overweight,"
but not obese], 82 c [PVD is a form of cardiovascular disease; see table
1.1], 83 d [PVD reduces the systolic blood pressure measured at the
ankle], 84 a [PVD patients need to exercise the affected region], 85 c
[continued aerobic exercise provides central cardiovascular adapta-
tions], 86 c [PVD patients should exercise at highest tolerable level to
achieve improvements; see table 10.1], 87 b [calculate workload in
kg·m·min⁻¹ as W times 6; calculate body mass in kg as lb/2.2; $\dot{V}O_2$
during leg cycling = 7 + 1.8(workload)/(body mass)], 88 a [net $\dot{V}O_2$ =
gross $\dot{V}O_2$ – 3.5; convert net $\dot{V}O_2$ in ml·min⁻¹·kg⁻¹ to L·min⁻¹; multiply $\dot{V}O_2$ in L·min⁻¹ by 5 to attain kcal·min⁻¹], 89 a [target $\dot{V}O_2$ = (fractional intensity)($\dot{V}O_2$max – 3.5) + 3.5; solve for workload in the following equation: $\dot{V}O_2$ during leg cycling = 7 + 1.8(workload)/(body
mass); calculate power in W as workload in kg·m·min⁻¹ divided by 6;
note: the answer is somewhat less than 50% of maximal power
because of the component for unloaded cycling in the $\dot{V}O_2$ equation],
90 d [beta-blockers reduce cardiac stimulation, thus reducing HR; also,
some beta-blockers have intrinsic *a*-adrenergic properties which can

result in peripheral vasoconstriction and thus decrease time to claudication]

Case Study A.10: 91 a [women who were not exercising prior to pregnancy should seek physician clearance to exercise], 92 d [supine exercise is contraindicated after the first trimester], 93 a [excessive heat may interfere with the closure of the neural tube during the first trimester], 94 d [exercise during pregnancy is generally safe for mother and fetus; one benign side effect is slightly lower birth weight], 95 b [there is little value in performing maximal exercise tests during pregnancy], 96 b [cardiovascular changes during pregnancy reduce the usefulness of HR and $\dot{V}O_2$ prescriptions], 97 c [exercise can be gradually increased throughout postpartum, but generally will not reach prepregnancy levels until 4-6 weeks], 98 d [exercise during pregnancy has many positive effects], 99 a [HRmax decreases and HRrest increases during pregnancy], 100 c [exercise may continue during the third trimester; nonweightbearing exercises may become easier and safer to perform]

Index

Note: Page numbers followed by *t* or *f* refer to the table or figure on that page.

1-RM
determining 84
and intensity of resistance training 23
and muscular strength and endurance 83
and resistance training for elderly 100
8-12 RM 83-84

A

ACE inhibitor 116
ACSM
approach to case studies 1
fitness components 10
norms 11
risk levels 2
screening questionnaire 3-4
ACSM guidelines 21
ACSM metabolic equations. *See* metabolic equations
ACSM recommendations
for duration of cardiovascular training 31
for resistance training 84
for resistance training for elderly 100-101
for training 21
for weight management 68
activities of daily living 98
adaptation to training 16-17
aerobic training 18
individual responses 20-21
resistance training 19
adipose tissue 67
ADL. *See* activities of daily living
adult-onset diabetes 123-124
case studies 131-137, 169-171
aerobic capacity 10
aerobic training
ACSM recommendations 21
adaptations 18
and fat loss 68
frequency of exercise 20, 30-32
for high school football player 150

sedentary client case study 92
time of exercise 30-32
type of exercise 29
aging and physical decline 97
angina 111
angioplasty 162
ankle swelling 4
antitachycardic pacemaker 118
arm cycling
metabolic equation 44
unloaded cycling term 58
$\dot{V}O_2$ case study 59
workload calculations 136
workload case study 60-61
arrhythmias 111
benefits of exercise against 112
types of pacemakers 117-118
arteries, peripheral vascular disease 139
arthritis 102, 160
aspirin 162
Åstrand, Per-Olaf 2
athletes
and fitness assessment 11
high school football player 150
ATP stores
response to aerobic training 18
response to resistance training 19
autonomic neuropathy 125

B

back stretch 82*f*
ballistic stretching 79
behavioral changes 14
bench press 86*f*
beta-blockers
and heart rate 39, 135
and hypertension 145
and peripheral vascular disease 172
biceps curl 88*f*
blood pressure. *See also* hypertension
ankle vs. brachial with PVD 140
benefits of exercise 112
and retinopathy 135

blood pressure *(continued)*
  during Valsalva maneuver 85
bodybuilder case study 93-96
body composition
  and fitness assessment 10
  hydrodensitometry 73
  methods for measuring 67
  and weight loss for novice bodybuilder 94
body fat. *See* weight loss
BodyGuard ergometer 56
body mass index (BMI)
  calculation 6
  and obesity 65
bone density 97, 98
Borg RPE scale. *See* Rating of Perceived
  Exertion (RPE) scale
bradycardia
  and pacemaker case study 164-167
  ventricular 117
breathing
  with chronic obstructive pulmonary
    disease (COPD) 144
  during resistance training 85
bronchitis, chronic 142-143

C

cadence, for stepping calculation 61
caffeine 39
calf raise 91*f*
caloric expenditure
  calculation for leg cycling 74-75
  calculation for post MI client 115
  calculation for treadmill running 72
  calculation for treadmill walking 71-72
  for client with type 2 diabetes 133-134
  and energy balance 66-67
  equivalent fat loss 75
  net and weight loss 68-69
  novice bodybuilder case study 95-96
  of running vs. walking 69-70
  with type 2 diabetes 130-131
  for walking 49
cancer, risk and inactivity 2
carbohydrates
  energy intake 66
  excess stored as fat 67
  intake prior to exercise with diabetes
    126
  intake to avoid hypoglycemia 127
cardiac output 18
cardiac rehabilitation 112-114
cardiac transplant 119-120
cardiorespiratory exercise prescription
  case study 31-32
  case study using %HRmax 35, 36
  for elderly 98-99
  for elderly, low fitness level 103-104
  frequency of exercise 30-32
  intensity and heart rate 33-39
  intensity of exercise 32-33
  interval training 33
  time of exercise 30-32
  type of exercise 29

using %HRR 37-38
using perceived exertion 39-40
using RPE and %HRR 40
by workload 41-42
cardizem 162
case studies
  ACSM approach to 1
  bodybuilder 93-96
  cardiac transplant 119-120
  cardiorespiratory exercise prescription
    31-32
  cardiorespiratory exercise prescription
    using %HRmax 35-36
  cardiorespiratory exercise prescription
    using %HRR 37-38
  cardiorespiratory exercise prescription
    using %HRR and RPE 40-41
  congestive heart failure 116-117
  elderly, high fitness 106-108
  elderly, low fitness 102-106
  high school football player 150
  hypertension 145-146
  myocardial infarction (MI) 114-116, 162-
    164
  older adult 160-162
  pacemaker 118-119, 164-167
  peripheral vascular disease 140-142,
    172-174
  pregnancy 174-176
  resistance training, sedentary client 91-93
  type 1 diabetes 128-130, 167-169
  type 2 diabetes 131-134, 169-171
  type 2 diabetes with complications 134-
    137
  using $\dot{V}O_2R$ 26-27
  using $\dot{V}O_2R$ and $\dot{V}O_2max$ 26-27
  $\dot{V}O_2$ for running 52-53
  $\dot{V}O_2$ for walking 48-49
  weight loss client 157-159
  weight loss using stationary bike 73-75
  weight loss using treadmill 70-73
  workload for running 53-55
  young adult, low risk 153-155
  young adult, moderate risk 155-156
cerebrovascular disease 2
children
  aerobic exercise prescription 148-149
  resistance training exercise prescription
    149-150
cholesterol 112
  hypercholesterolemia case study 6, 7, 9
chronic bronchitis 142-143
chronic obstructive pulmonary disease
  (COPD)
  benefits of exercise 142-143
  case study 143-144
  and peripheral vascular disease 140-142
  pursed-lip breathing 144
chronotropic incompetence 165
cigarette smoking
  and ACSM risk levels 2
  cessation and risk 7
  and chronic obstructive pulmonary
    disease 142-143

circulation. *See* peripheral vascular disease
claudication scale 141
concentric phase 83
congestive heart failure 111, 116
  case study 116-117
conversion of units
  kg·m·min^{-1} to watts 57-58
  mph to running pace 54
  oxygen consumption to caloric
    expenditure 49
  speed 48, 49
  table 46-47
  weight 48
COPD. *See* chronic obstructive pulmonary
  disease
coronary artery disease 111
  as complication for diabetes 135
  and diabetes mellitus 125
coronary heart disease
  pain from ischemia 4
  risk and inactivity 2
CP stores
  response to aerobic training 18
  response to resistance training 19
criterion standards 11
curl-ups 89*f*
cycle ergometry. *See also* leg cycling
  flywheel revolution distance 55-56
  work rate equation 55

D

DDDR pacemaker 118, 165
defibrillators 111
delayed-onset muscle soreness (DOMS)
  and resistance training 87
  and resistance training for elderly 101
detraining 16*f*, 17*f*, 20
diabetes
  case study for type 1 128-130, 167-169
  case study for type 2 131-134, 169-171
  case study for type 2 with complications
    134-137
  in children 148
  exercise prescription for type 1 125-128
  glucose tolerance test 124
  increase in incidence 65
  medical evaluation prior to exercise 125
  risk and inactivity 2
  types of 123
diabetic coma 127
diuretic 116
dizziness
  and ACSM risk levels 4
  and risk stratification 10
DOMS. *See* delayed-onset muscle soreness
duration of exercise. *See* time of exercise
dyspnea 117
  and COPD 143
  and exercise intensity 120
  scale 144

E

eccentric phase 83
echocardiography 116

ejection fraction 114
  after myocardial infarction 162
  and congestive heart failure 116
elderly
  adaptation to training 98
  cardiorespiratory exercise prescription
    98-99
  case study 160-162
  high fitness case study 106-108
  low fitness case study 102-106
  resistance training 100-102
emphysema 142-143
endurance. *See* aerobic capacity; muscular
  endurance
energy balance 66-67
energy expenditure. *See also* metabolic
  equations
  and fat loss 69
essential hypertension 144-145
ethyl alcohol 66
exercise and risk 2
exercise prescription. *See also* cardiorespiratory exercise prescription; resistance training
  ACSM guidelines 22*t*
  for fat loss 68-70
  and goal setting 14

F

fat
  conversion of excess carbohydrate and
    protein 67
  energy intake 66
fatigue
  and overload 16
  as symptom of ventricular bradycardia
    118
fat loss. *See* weight loss
fat metabolism
  equivalent caloric expenditure 75
  response to aerobic training 18
fitness, changing definitions of 77
fitness components 10
fitness level, and intensity of cardiovascular training 32-33
FITT principle 21
  for cardiac rehabilitation 112-114
  and hypertension 145-146
  for inpatient cardiac rehabilitation 113
  for outpatient cardiac rehabilitation 113-
    114
  with peripheral vascular disease 140-141
flexibility. *See also* stretching exercises
  definition 77-78
  and fitness assessment 10
flexibility training
  ACSM recommendations 21
  after cardiovascular training 30
  for elderly, high fitness case study 108
  for elderly, low fitness case study 106
  frequency of exercise 20
  intensity of exercise 23
  stretching technique 78-82

flywheel revolution distance
    for BodyGuard ergometer 56
    for Monark arm ergometer 59
    for Monark leg ergometer 55
    for Tunturi ergometer 56
frequency of exercise
    ACSM recommendations 22*t*
    for aerobic training 20
    for cardiorespiratory exercise prescription 30-32
    and detraining 17*f*
    and FITT principle 21
    flexibility training 20
    and overtraining 17*f*
    for resistance training 83
    for weight management 68

G

gestational diabetes mellitus 124
    exercise prescription 131
glucose
    interpreting value prior to exercise 128
    level for diabetes diagnosis 124
    monitoring during exercise with diabetes 126
    post-exercise value 127
    and types of diabetes 123
glucose tolerance test 124
glycogen stores
    and caloric intake 67
    response to aerobic training 18
    response to resistance training 19
goal setting 12-14
    and exercise prescription 14
graded exercise test 35
gravity, correcting for 47

H

hamstring stretch 81*f*
HDL, and hypercholesterolemia 7
heart attack. *See* myocardial infarction (MI)
heart disease
    benefits of exercise 112
    cardiac transplant 119-120
    congestive heart failure case study 116-117
    coronary ischemia and Valsalva maneuver 85
    and ejection fraction 114
    myocardial infarction (MI) 114-116
    myocardial infarction (MI) case study 162-164
    pacemaker case study 118-119
    types of 111
heart rate
    and beta-blockers 39
    changes during pregnancy 147
    and intensity of cardiovascular training 33-39
    and medications 39
    relationship to oxygen consumption 33
heart rate reserve
    case study 94-95

    definition 21-22
    and equivalent exercise intensities 22*t*
    error introduced by $\dot{V}O_2$max 23
    relationship to $\dot{V}O_2$max 24*f*
    relationship to $\dot{V}O_2R$ 25*f*
    and target heart rate 37-39
heat sensitivity
    in children 149
    during pregnancy 147
high-risk
    ACSM definition 2
    case study 9-10
HRR. *See* heart rate reserve
Humalog 128
    timing of dosage while exercising 129
hydration
    for children while exercising 149
    for pregnant women while exercising 147
hydrodensitometry 73
hypercholesterolemia 6, 7, 9
hyperglycemia 125
hyperlipidemia. *See* cholesterol
hypertension 144
hypoglycemia
    avoiding while exercising with diabetes 126
    medication while exercising 171
    steps to avoid 127
    symptoms 126
    and type 1 diabetes 167
    and type 2 diabetes 131
hypokinetic diseases 65
hypothermia 149

I

ICD pacemaker 118
immunosuppressive drug therapy 120
impaired fasting glucose (IFG) 124
    exercise prescription 131
impaired glucose tolerance (IGT) 124
    exercise prescription 131
inactivity
    diseases associated with 2
    and hypertension 145
    and insulin sensitivity 123
    and obesity 67
insulin
    intake prior to exercise with diabetes 126
    intermediate-acting 128
    response to aerobic training 18
    sensitivity and exercise 124
    short-acting (Humalog) 128
    timing of dosage while exercising 129
    and types of diabetes 123
insulin-dependent diabetes mellitus (IDDM) 123
intensity of exercise
    ACSM recommendations 22*t*
    calculation for elderly, low fitness case study 104-105
    and caloric expenditure 72

for cardiorespiratory exercise prescription 32-33
for cardiovascular fitness in elderly 99
difference from speed of exercise 36
equivalents using %HRR, %$\dot{V}O_2$R, and %$\dot{V}O_2$max 22t
and FITT principle 21
with pacemaker 118-119
and perceived exertion 39-40
predictable and variable 41
relationship to duration of cardiovascular training 31
for resistance training 23, 83
and talk test 39
and $\dot{V}O_2$R 23-26
for weight management 68
intermediate-acting insulin (NPH) 128
timing of dosage while exercising 129
interval training 33
ischemic leg pain. *See* peripheral vascular disease
isolation during resistance training 84-85

J

joints. *See* flexibility
juvenile-onset diabetes 123

K

K+ supplement 116
Karvonen method 37-39
for patient with pacemaker 118-119
ketosis 126
kilocalories. *See* caloric expenditure
kilograms, conversion to 47

L

lactate threshold
and adaptations of elderly 98
response to aerobic training 18
lactic acid
and peripheral vascular disease 139
and warm-down 30
lat pull-down 87f
LDL cholesterol, and hypercholesterolemia 7
left ventricle
response to aerobic training 18
response to resistance training 19
leg curl 90f
leg cycling
metabolic equation 44
unloaded cycling term 55
$\dot{V}O_2$ case study 56-57
weight loss case study 73-75
workload case study 57-58
leg extension 90f
leg pain. *See* peripheral vascular disease
low-risk
ACSM definition 2
case studies 7-8
and exercise recommendations 5

M

maximum heart rate
and %$\dot{V}O_2$R 34t
case study 35
estimating 34-35
during pregnancy 147
and target heart rate 33-37
measurements, conversion of units table 46-47t
medications
ACE inhibitor 116
aspirin 162
beta-blockers 39, 135, 145, 172
cardizem 162
diuretic 116
hypoglycemic 171
immunosuppressive drug therapy 120
K+ supplement 116
for obesity 68
Pentoxifylline 172
and training principles for elderly 98
metabolic equations 44
conversion of units 45
conversion of units table 46-47t
listed 44
modifications to 43-44
purposes 44-45
$\dot{V}O_2$ for arm cycling 59-60
$\dot{V}O_2$ for leg cycling 56-57
$\dot{V}O_2$ for running 52-53
$\dot{V}O_2$ for stepping 61-62
$\dot{V}O_2$ for walking 48-49
workload for arm cycling 60-61
workload for leg cycling 57-58
workload for running 53-55
workload for walking 49-51
metabolism
in children 149
and diabetes mellitus 125
resting, and MET levels 42
METs
definition 41
and equivalent exercise intensities 22t
requirement for phase III/IV cardiac rehabilitation 113
and resting metabolism 42
for running 52-53
for unloaded cycling 55
MI. *See* myocardial infarction (MI)
mitochondria 18
mode of exercise. *See* type of exercise
moderate risk
ACSM definition 2
case study 5-7
and exercise recommendations 5
Monark ergometer
arm cycling 136-137
flywheel revolution distance, arm 59
leg cycling 55
motor unit recruitment 19
muscle, response to resistance training 19
muscle soreness
and proprioceptive neuromuscular facilitation 80

muscle soreness *(continued)*
  and resistance training 87
  and resistance training for elderly 101
muscular endurance
  definition 83
  and fitness assessment 10
muscular strength. *See also* resistance
    training
  and adaptations of elderly 98
  and aging 97
  definition 83
  and fitness assessment 10
  and neural recruitment patterns 19
myocardial infarction (MI) 111
  case study 162-164
myoglobin 18

N

neck stretch 79*f*
nephropathy 125
neural recruitment patterns 19
neurological complications of diabetes 125
nicotine 39
noninsulin-dependent diabetes 123-124
norms
  and goal setting 12
  limitations of 11
NPH. *See* intermediate-acting insulin
    (NPH)

O

obesity
  ACSM classification 6
  and benefits of exercise 112
  and body mass index 6
  causes of 67
  in children 148
  criteria for 9
  and hypertension 145
  and insulin sensitivity 123
  prevalence of 65
older adult. *See* elderly
orthopedic issues
  arthritis 102, 160
  and weightbearing exercise 99
osteoporosis
  and exercise recommendations 99
  risk and inactivity 2
overheating
  and children 149
  during pregnancy 147
overload 15
  and resistance training 83
overload principle 16-17
overtraining 16*f*, 17*f*, 20
oxygen consumption
  for arm cycling 59
  conversion to caloric expenditure 49
  as format to metabolic equations 44
  gross vs. net 45
  and intensity of exercise 32
  for leg cycling 56-57
  from metabolic equations 44
  and MET levels 41

quantifying during exercise 41
  relationship to heart rate 33
  for running 52-53
  for stepping 61-62
  for unloaded cycling 55
  use with special populations 117
  for walking 48-49
oxygen saturation, and COPD 143

P

pace, calculation for running 53-55
pacemakers 111
  case study 164-167
  types of 117-118
pancreas 123
Pentoxifylline 172
perceived exertion 39-40
  case study 40
  use with cardiac transplant patient 120
percutaneous transluminal coronary
    angioplasty (PTCA) 114, 162
periodization 18
peripheral edema 116
peripheral neuropathy 125
  case study 134-137
peripheral vascular disease (PVD) 139
  case study 140-142, 172-174
  claudication scale 141
platelet stickiness 112
PNF. *See* proprioceptive neuromuscular
    facilitation
population norms 11
potassium supplement 116
pounds, conversion to kilograms 47
power
  conversion of units of measure 47
  readout for cycle ergometers 56
pregnancy
  case study 146-147, 174-176
  exercise prescription 146
  and gestational diabetes mellitus 124
primary hypertension 144-145
progression 17-18
proprioceptive neuromuscular facilitation
  definition 23
  technique 79-80
protein, excess stored as fat 67
pulmonary edema 116
pulse oximeter 143
pursed-lip breathing 144

Q

quadriceps
  leg extension exercise 90*f*
  stretching 80

R

range of motion. *See also* flexibility
  and flexibility 77-78
  and intensity of flexibility training 23
  during resistance training 84
rate-responsive pacemakers 118
Rating of Perceived Exertion (RPE) scale
    39

case study 40
and hypertension 146
and pregnancy 147
for resistance training for elderly 100
reciprocal inhibition 81
recovery
  individual variability 21
  and overload 16
  and periodization 18
  and training principles 20
resistance training
  ACSM recommendations 21, 84
  adaptations 19
  for cardiac rehabilitation 112
  for children 149-150
  concentric phase 83
  determining 8-12 RM 83-84
  eccentric phase 83
  for elderly 100-102
  for elderly, high fitness case study 108
  for elderly, low fitness case study 105-106
  and fat loss 68
  guidelines 83-84
  for high school football player 150
  intensity of exercise 23
  negative repetitions 86-87
  novice bodybuilder case study 93-96
  program for sedentary client 91-93
  and specificity principle 19
  spotting technique 85-87
  sticking point 87
  technique 84-85
resistance training exercises
  bench press 86f
  biceps curl 88f
  calf raise 91f
  curl-ups 89f
  lat pull-down 87f
  leg curl 90f
  leg extension 90f
  squats 89f
  triceps extension 88f
resting heart rate
  for elderly 99
  and intensity of cardiovascular training 36
  during pregnancy 147
resting metabolism
  addition to stepping equation 44
  and energy balance 66
  and MET levels 42, 52
  and percent body fat 67
  in stepping calculation 61
retinopathy
  case study 134-137
  and diabetes mellitus 125
risk
  ACSM levels 2
  after smoking cessation 7
  associated with exercise 2
  determining from ACSM questionnaire 4
  and goal setting 12
risk stratification case studies
  female executive 9
  female sales consultant 7-8

male college student 9-10
male construction worker 5-7
male public school teacher 8
ROM. See range of motion
RPE. See Rating of Perceived Exertion (RPE) scale
running
  caloric expenditure vs. walking 69-70
  metabolic equation 44
  vertical component 51-52
  VO_2 case study 52-53
  workload case study 53-55

S

salt and hypertension 145
S_aO_2 143
screening 2-5
  ACSM questionnaire 3-4
secondary hypertension 144-145
serotonin inhibitors 68
smoking. See cigarette smoking
specificity principle 19
speed
  calculation for running 53-55
  calculation for treadmill running 115
  and caloric expenditure 72
  conversion from kph to m·min^{-1} 46
  conversion of units 48
  difference from intensity of exercise 36
  during resistance training 85
  of walking with training in elderly 98
squats 89f
standards, norms vs. criterion referenced data 11
static stretching 78
stationary bike. See leg cycling
ST depression 134
stepping
  metabolic equation 44
  modification to equation 61
  VO_2 case study 61-62
  workload case study 62-63
sticking point 87
strength. See muscular strength
strength training. See resistance training
stress test 5
stretching exercises
  back hyperextension 82f
  hamstring 81f
  neck 79f
  quadriceps 80f
  reciprocal inhibition 81
  safest time for 78
  sit-and-twist 82f
  types of 78
swimming 41
sympathomimetics 68
systolic blood pressure (SBP) with pacemaker 116-117

T

tachycardia 118
talk test 39
  for elderly, low fitness case study 103

target heart rate
  calculating by % HRmax 33-37
  calculating by % HRR (Karvonen
    method) 37-39
  calculation for post MI client 115
  for cardiac transplant patient 120
  for client with type 1 diabetes 129
  for client with type 2 diabetes 132-133
  for elderly high fitness case study 107-108
  for elderly, low fitness case study 103-104
  for patient with pacemaker 116-117
    with peripheral vascular disease 142
  sample calculation 74
  for type 2 diabetes with complications
    135-136
  use with pacemakers 117-118
thermic effect of food 66, 67
time of exercise
  ACSM recommendations 22t
  for cardiorespiratory exercise prescrip-
    tion 30-32
  and FITT principle 21
  for resistance training 83
  for weight management 68
tobacco 2
training, definition 17
training principles 15-16
  detraining 20
  overload 16-17
  overtraining 20
  progression 17-18
  recovery 20
  specificity 19
transplant. See cardiac transplant
treadmill walking
  caloric expenditure 71-72
  grade 49-51
triceps extension 88f
trunk stretch 82f
Tunturi ergometer 56
type of exercise
  ACSM recommendations 22t
  for cardiorespiratory exercise prescrip-
    tion 29
  for cardiorespiratory exercise prescrip-
    tion for elderly 99
  and FITT principle. See time of exercise
  predictable and variable 41
  for resistance training for elderly 101

U
underwater weighing 73
units of measure
  conversion table 46-47t
  for oxygen consumption 45
unloaded cycling 43, 55
  for arm cycling 58
uphill walking and running 51-52

V
Valsalva maneuver 85
  and hypertension 146
  and retinopathy 135
ventilation, response to aerobic training 18
ventilatory threshold 120
ventricular bradycardias 117

case study 118-119
vertical component of walking and
  running 51-52
$\dot{V}O_2$. See oxygen consumption
$\dot{V}O_2$max
  and adaptations of elderly 98
  and beta-blockers 145
  and equivalent exercise intensities 22t
  error between %HRR 23
  and fitness assessment 10
  with peripheral vascular disease 142
  relationship to heart rate reserve 24f
$\dot{V}O_2R$
  and %HRmax values 34t
  case study using 26-27
  concept explained 23-26
  definition 23
  and equivalent exercise intensities 22t
  formula 26
  and intensity of cardiovascular training 32
  relationship to heart rate reserve 25f
  sample calculation 27
VVI pacemaker 117
VVIR pacemaker 118

W
walking
  caloric expenditure vs. running 69-70
  as cardiovascular exercise for elderly 99
  energy cost 48
  metabolic equation 44
  vertical component 51-52
  $\dot{V}O_2$ case study 48-49
  workload case study 49-51
warm-down
  after cardiovascular training 30
  stretching during 78
warm-up 30-32
watt 56
  calculation case study 57-58
weightbearing activity 99
weightlifting. See resistance training
weight loss
  ACSM guidelines 67-68
  case study 157-159
  case study using stationary bike 73-75
  case study using treadmill 70-73
  for client with type 2 diabetes 132
  and energy balance 66-67
  exercise prescription 68-70
  leg cycling calculations for 56-57
  for novice bodybuilder 94
  with type 2 diabetes 130-131
weight management (gain) 150
workload
  for arm cycling 60-61
  for arm ergometer 136
  for client with type 2 diabetes 133
  and intensity of cardiovascular training
    41-42
  for leg cycling 57-58
  from metabolic equations 45
  for running 53-55
  for stepping 62-63
  vertical component 51-52
  for walking 49-51

About the Authors

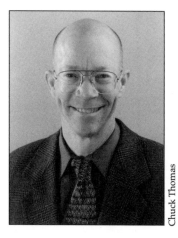

Chuck Thomas

David P. Swain, PhD, has been an exercise science researcher and educator for more than 15 years. He is a professor of exercise physiology at Old Dominion University. Dr. Swain is a certified Program Director for the ACSM, and he has served as a Health/Fitness Instructor workshop director for eight years. The ACSM named him a Fellow in 1986. Dr. Swain authored the key research studies that established the use of $\dot{V}O_2$ reserve for exercise prescription adopted by the ACSM; and he authored the recent revisions to the organization's metabolic calculations for determining the oxygen consumption of various modes of exercise in the Metabolic Calculations appendix in *ACSM's Guidelines for Exercise Testing and Prescription*, sixth edition.

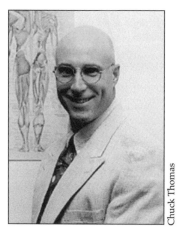

Chuck Thomas

Brian C. Leutholtz, PhD, is an associate professor of exercise physiology at Old Dominion University, where he is director of the Therapeutic Exercise Program for Chronic Diseases. Dr. Leutholtz is a Fellow of and certified Program Director for the ACSM. He is the author of several recent books and workbooks on exercise and disease management.

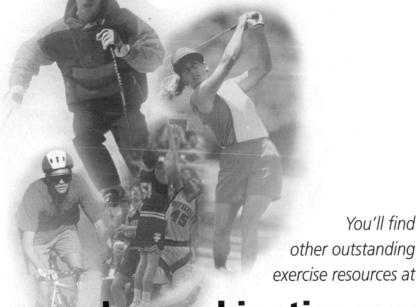